ARCTIC ROOT

(RHODIOLA ROSEA)

ARCTIC ROOT

(RHODIOLA ROSEA)

THE POWERFUL NEW GINSENG ALTERNATIVE

CARL GERMANO, R.D. C.N.S. L.D.N.

AND

ZAKIR RAMAZANOV, PH.D.

WITH MARIA DEL MAR BERNAL SUAREZ, PH.D.

EDITING BY BRIAN APPELL, B.S.

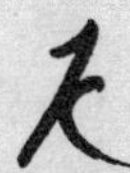

KENSINGTON BOOKS

KENSINGTON PUBLISHING CORP.

http://www.kensingtonbooks.com

This book is designed to provide accurate and authoritative information in regard to the subject matter covered. It is sold with the understanding that the publisher is not engaged in rendering medical or related professional services and that without personal consultation the authors cannot and do not render judgment or advice about a particular patient or medical condition. If medical advice is required, the services of a competent professional should be sought. While every attempt has been made to provide accurate information, the author and publisher cannot be held responsible for any errors or omissions.

KENSINGTON BOOKS are published by

Kensington Publishing Corp.
850 Third Avenue
New York, NY 10022

First Printing: May, 1999
10 9 8 7 6 5 4 3 2 1

Printed in the United States of America

CONTENTS

INTRODUCTION

For thousands of years, certain civilizations, notably, the Chinese, Egyptians, Indians, and Russians have revered herbal remedies for their beneficial healing properties. But in many countries, especially the United States, twentieth century medicine has put herbal healing on the back burner, making pharmaceuticals the primary form of medical treatment. In the last decade, however, renewed interest in alternative therapies and preventative health care has brought attention back to herbs and their beneficial active ingredients. Today, research studies published in reputable medical journals, such as *The Journal of the American Medical Association,* have pointed to the complementary role that herbs play in treating disease. Yet, of all the benefits herbs are noted for, the ability of an herb to help the body adapt to stress, improve performance, and increase resistance to disease is of most importance. Essentially, we are describing the activity of the class of herbs known as adaptogens. While ginseng has received all the attention as an adaptogen, the use of Rhodiola rosea (Arctic root) by the Russians has shown this herb to go above and beyond ginseng. The scientifc work on Rhodiola rosea's active components in addressing heart disease, cancer/immunity, and performance (mental and physical) is impressive and places Rhodiola rosea as one of the most important herbs and greatest gifts bestowed upon us.

The Chinese described adaptogens as ''superior'' plants being completely harmless to the body while exerting profound supportive effects. Adaptogens work by activating the basic and vital functions of the body to help it remain healthy under unflavorable conditions—making the body able to **adapt.** Essentially, the ability for the body to adapt to unfavorable biological, chemical, and psychological conditions provides an effective defense and means for survival. Rsearch into adaptogens is on the increase, and many scientists are unraveling the benefits of these medicinal plants as profound contributors to our health and well-being.

With the Cold War behind us, Russian scientists have blessed us with a wealth of information on one of the most important adaptogens: Rhodiola rosea. It is our intention to provide you with the history of Rhodiola and scientific evidence that exists on this plant's marvelous active ingredients. As you read through this book, you will soon understand the important contribution that Rhodiola may have on our heart, immune system, and ability to perform (physically and psychologically), as it increases our resistance to stress and disease.

CHAPTER 1

Stress: An Old Friend Turned New Enemy

Stress: An Old Friend Turned New Enemy

Let's play a game. When I say a word you tell me the first thing that comes to your mind. Alright, let's start. **STRESS!** If you're like the many millions in today's fast-paced and quick-tempered society, no doubt the word "stress" stirred up negative feelings and thoughts. Stress is a buzzword tossed around with abandon by the media, medical and scientific communities, and the general public. It is the *primus inter pares* of excuses and explanations for everything from headaches to mental breakdown, and that designation isn't too far from the truth when we examine stress' effects in the body. In fact, it may be worse. Stress, however, is not a new concept endemic to industrialized countries. In fact, it is a process older than our species and, in some respects, has played an integral part in our development.

Stress is any factor imposed on the organism that disrupts the normal biochemical and physiological equilibrium and requires a response that affects the organism. It is the response of the body to any demand whether it is physical, emotional, environmental, and/or chemical. In its most basic form, stress is the "fight or flight" response that is innately coded into every living organism. In early man, this response protected us from imminent danger, such as the attack of a wild beast or a rival clan. Man either stood his ground or ran for safer ground. Whether he fought or fled, it was necessary to prepare him quickly for the event. That job fell predominantly to two important systems involved in the stress response—the sympathetic nervous system and the adrenal glands.

Sympathetic Nervous System: Jump-starting the Stress Response

The sympathetic nervous system (SNS) is one half of the autonomic nervous system (ANS), a division of the nervous system that regulates many systems in the body. Without it, most of our day would be spent sitting around mentally adjusting our heart rate or blood pressure or digestive processes; truly, a life less lived. By working at the subconscious level, the ANS takes care of all these processes, so we don't have to think about them. Heart rate, blood pressure, expenditure of metabolic energy, smooth muscle contraction, and relaxation, glandular activity and gastrointestinal motility all fall under the auspices of the ANS.

The other half of the autonomic nervous system is called the parasympathetic nervous system (you guessed it—PNS). Both the SNS and PNS are critical for the body to adapt to an ever-changing environment, and the stimulation of one usually antagonizes the other. The parasympathetic nervous system enhances activities that gain and conserve energy. Stimulation of digestion and a decrease in heart rate assures that energy stores are increasing while expenditure is not. Contrary to the PNS, the sympathetic nervous system increases energy expenditure and prepares an individual for action. It is the sympathetic nervous system that plays a major role in the stress response. It is also this branch of the autonomic nervous system that may contribute to the damaging effects resulting from stress.

During normal situations, the primary function of the sympathetic nervous system is to counteract the activity of the parasympathetic nervous system just enough to carry out normal processes requiring energy. During times of stress however, the SNS dominates.

The immediate and acute reactions following exposure to a stressor is the result of SNS stimulation:

- Pupils dilate
- Heart rate, force of contraction and blood pressure, increases
- Blood vessels in nonessential organs constrict, while blood vessels in the systems involved in the stress response dilate. This reaction assures an adequate blood supply for the latter.
- Bronchial tubes in the lungs dilate, while rapid, deeper breathing is initiated, allowing a faster movement of oxygen in and out of the lungs.
- Energy reserves are mobilized, increasing blood sugar and fatty acid levels.

Acute stress is promptly and effectively addressed by the sympathetic nervous system. But prolonged exposure to stress requires a backup system, which is where the adrenal glands come in. See Table 1.1 for a summary of SNS' effects.

The Adrenal Glands: Turbochargers in the Stress Response

Think of it this way: Imagine the human body as an automobile engine. The gas pedal would represent the SNS, providing more energy for us to work harder.

Table 1.1 Effects of the SNS on the Body

Effects of the SNS on the Body
Pupils Dilate
Salivation Is Inhibited
Bronchiolar Relaxes
Heart Rate Increases
Gastric Activity Decreases
Hepatic Glucose Release Increases
Catecholamine Releases
Bladder Relaxes
Sexual Activity Decreases

But the accelerator only goes to the floor. In order to go faster, we need a turbocharger to "kick in," providing more energy and power. Our body doesn't have one turbocharger but two—the adrenal glands which sit astride each kidney and release the hormones collectively termed catecholamines. Derived from the amino acid tyrosine, epinephrine (adrenaline) and norepinephrine (noradrenaline) are the principal catecholamines (Figures 1.1 and 1.2). Like the SNS, epinephrine and norepinephrine primarily act by causing vasoconstriction, increased heart rate and forced contraction, increased oxygen consumption, and bronchial dilation. The catecholamines are catabolic in their effects, mobi-

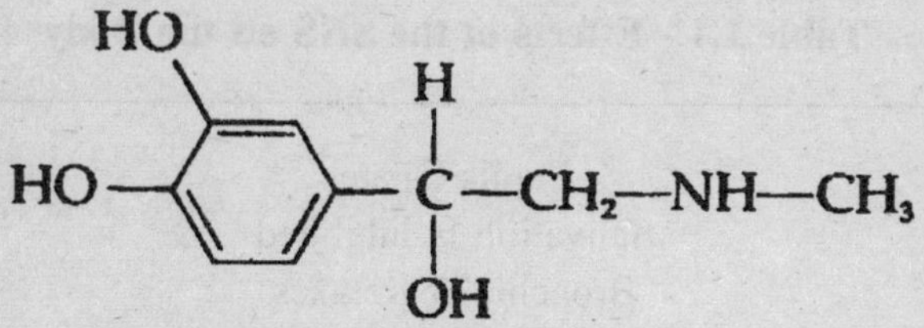

HO

HO — C — CH_2 — NH — CH_3 (H above C; OH below C)

OH

Figure 1.1 Epinephrine (Adrenaline)

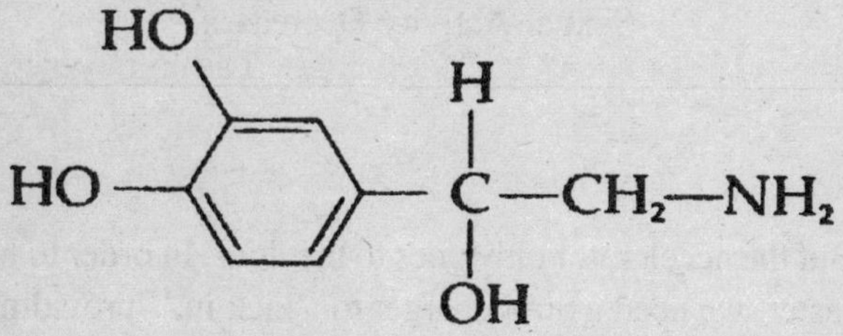

HO

HO — C — CH_2 — NH_2 (H above C; OH below C)

OH

Figure 1.2 Norepinephrine

lizing stored glucose in the liver and skeletal muscles and fatty acids from adipose tissue. Together, catecholamines and the SNS are a synergistic power pack, enhancing the stress response.

In addition to sympathetic nervous system stimulation and catecholamine release, additional compounds, called corticosteroids, are also synthesized in the adrenal glands and released into circulation during the stress response. Corticosteroids are divided into two general categories: glucocorticoids and mineralcorticoids.

Cortisone, cortisol (hydrocortisone), and corticosterone are classified as glucocorticoids. The name glucocorticoids reflects the primary action of these hormones, metabolism of carbohydrates, particularly glucose and proteins. Cortisol is the most abundant and most active of all glucocorticoids and plays a crucial role in regulating metabolism during stress (Figure 1.3). The release of cortisol into circulation ensures that an adequate level of adenosine triphosphate (ATP—the cells' "energy molecule") is maintained in the body. It does this by increasing glucose, fatty acid, and amino acid metabolism to support ATP production.

The mineralcorticoids are so named because of their ability to influence mineral balance, particularly sodium and potassium. Aldosterone (Figure 1.4), the most famous and biologically active of the mineralcorticoids, acts on the kidneys to increase sodium reabsorption while at the same time expediting potassium's excretion. The combined effect of potassium loss and sodium retention is increased fluid volume and blood pressure. Mineralcorticoids are mobilized during the stress response to maintain fluid volume and prevent dehydration and low blood pressure. As we will see later, during prolonged stressful conditions, these processes lead to changes in the organism that ultimately result in the impairment of health. But more on that later. See Table 1.2 for a summary of the stress hormones.

In primordial man, the stress response was a survival tool. When the danger passed, the multitude of chemicals released by the body to prepare for the stress were safely detoxified until they were called for again. Two events in man's history, however, were about to change all that: technology and civilization.

Civilization: A Catalyst for Change

Soon, man found himself cluttered and confined within cities. He found himself trying to survive in a new environment that evolution had not prepared him for. With the exponential advances in technology and civilization, man's lagging evolutionary adaptation left

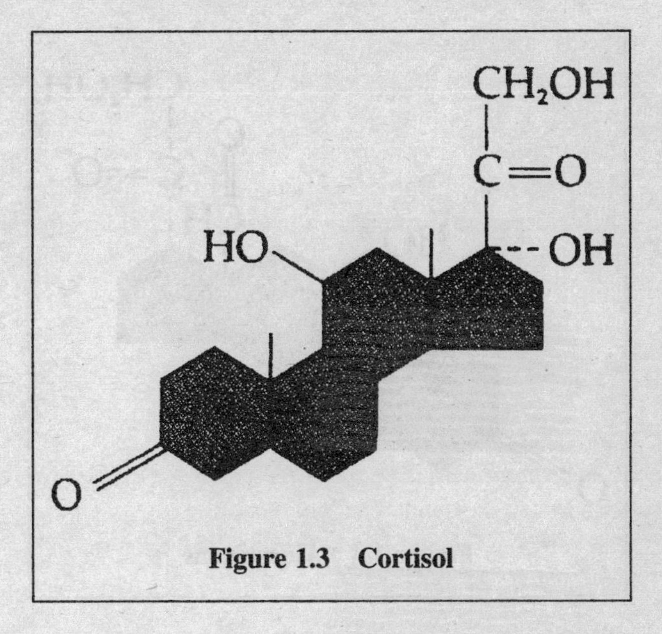

Figure 1.3 Cortisol

him ill-prepared for the new type of stresses that inundated him. Instead of fighting for his life, man faced new enemies in the form of environmental pollution, toxins in our air, water, and food; the emotional headwaters we swim through every day; and economic, family, and social responsibilities. Unfortunately, our ability to adapt to stress is further hampered by our diets of processed and refined convenience foods, devoid of nutrients needed to protect us from stress.

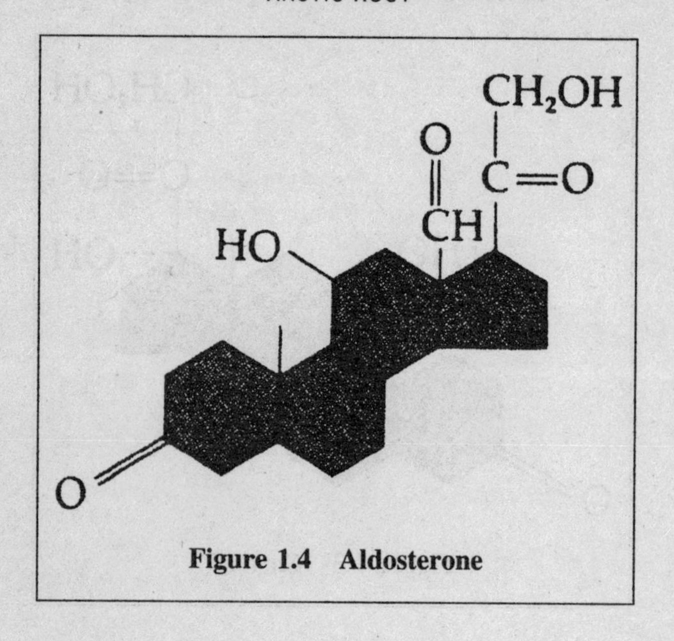

Figure 1.4 Aldosterone

Unlike early man, who dealt with stress periodically throughout the day, modern man's experience with stress is more chronic in nature, far more insidious and devastating to the human system. Doctor Hans Selye, world-renowned for his studies of stress on an organism, recognized the impact that long-term stress has and conceived what is known as ''The General Adaptation Syndrome'' (GAS). Doctor Selye divided GAS into three phases:

Table 1.2 The Stress Chemicals

Catecholamines
Adrenaline (epinephrine)
Noradrenaline (norepinephrine)

Glucocorticoids
Cortisone
Hydrocortisone
Corticosterone

Mineralcorticoids
Aldosterone

1. ''Alarm''—Organism experiences a heightened activity of the sympathetic nervous system and increased corticosteroid and catecholamine release. The weight of the thymus, spleen, lymph glands, and liver diminish while the weight of the adrenal glands increases. The alarm phase is characterized by a state of degenerative breakdown in the organism.
2. ''Resistance''—If the stressor continues, the organism responds with a heightened resistance

to the damaging factors. Anabolic functions prevail over catabolic processes, and the organism becomes increasingly resistant to the stressor.

3. "Exhaustion"—With the continuing assault of the stressor, the resistance built up in phase two is lost. The organism is no longer able to resist the stressor.

Disease and conditions associated with stress manifest themselves in the exhaustion phase. Considering that 80 percent of all illnesses are reported to have their roots in stress, it appears that most of us live in "exhaustion." The major killers in today's society—cancer, heart disease, stroke, hypertension, and diabetes—can be all traced to stress. What's worse, the exposure to one form of stress seems to diminish our resistance to other forms, a type of synergistic "one-two punch." It would seem that stress, once a beneficial tool for human survival, is now killing us from the inside.

There is hope, however. Nature has bestowed upon us a collection of plants that can effectively combat the effects of stress and return us to our birthright: our health. Although eradicating stress from our life seems impossible, we can respond by diminishing its effects. Enter adaptogens, and in particular Rhodiola rosea, nature's answer to stress.

In the chapters that follow, we take a closer look at stress and the role that it plays in disease. The public is demanding effective and safe answers to disease, and scientists are working to understand its mechanisms and causative factors. As scientists strive to understand the nature of disease, nature itself offers a remarkable plant with the ability to effectively combat stress, improve performance, and prevent disease. The plant is Rhodiola rosea.

CHAPTER 2

Rhodiola rosea: Adaptogens—Nature's Solution to Sickness

Adaptogens: Nature's Solution to Sickness

The science of nutrition is a young science. It is only within the past several decades that interest has developed in the various components of food, and the roles they play in the body. As researchers extracted and isolated in their tests and experiments they uncovered many of the vitamins that we are familiar with today. In fact, the science of chemistry has discovered that minerals and vitamins play a life and death role in the functioning of the body. Recently as well, public awareness of these nutrients has grown substantially both by our efforts to achieve optimum health and as reflected in the growth of the natural products industry. Although vitamins and minerals have shared the spotlight for importance, a new class of nutrients is emerging as equally important. This new class of nutrients is called "phytonutrients"—powerful compounds found in plants that have profound beneficial effects on the body.

When the former Soviet Union opened its iron curtain to the West, adaptogens, and their diverse benefits, were unveiled. So potent are these adaptogens that they may, one day, share the spotlight with vitamins and minerals—they're that important. It is necessary, however, to understand which plants are true adaptogens. To be considered an adaptogen, a plant must conform to the following criteria:

- The plant must be nontoxic and totally harmless to the body. It must allow the continuing normal physiological functioning of the individual.
- The action it exerts must be nonspecific and should maintain normal body functions despite a wide range of onslaughts to the body (i.e., stress).
- It should normalize body functions irrespective of existing pathological condition.

As you can see, this is a tall order for one substance. Unlike drugs which carry with them the possibility of side effects, adaptogens must benefit the body without disturbing it or doing it any harm. Not many plants possess adaptogenic properties, and if it weren't for Soviet scientists, the adaptogenic qualities of Rhodiola

Table 2.1 Adaptogenic Plants

Andrographis paniculata *(Acanthaceae)*
Arogyappcha *(Trichopus zeylanicus)*
Ashwaganda *(Withania somnifera)*
Chickpea *(Cicer arietinum)*
Chinese magnolia *(Schizandra chinensis)*
Dangshen *(Codonopis pilosula)*
Ginseng *(Panax ginseng)*
Golden root *(Rhodiola rosea)*
Hoppea dichotoma *(Gentianaceae)*
Leuzea carthamoides
Maral root *(Rhaponticum carthamoides)*
Reishi *(Ganoderma lucidum)*
Siberian ginseng *(Eleutherococcus senticosus)*
Tulsi *(Ocimum sanctum)*

rosea and other plants might never have been discovered (Table 2.1).

Serious research on adaptogens began in 1947 under the auspices of Dr. Nicole Laserev from the Vladivostock branch of the Far-East Academy of Sciences. He reported on several indigenous plants that helped increase the body's natural resistance to environmental stresses and later coined the term "adaptogens." Later, a student of Dr. Lasarev and perhaps the best known of these pioneers, Dr. Israel Brekhman, brought adaptogens to the attention of the world. Brekhman's pioneering work with adaptogens, in fact, was the impetus behind their fame in both the Soviet Union and then throughout the world.

While in medical school, Dr. Brekhman's initial exposure to adaptogens occurred while participating in experiments designed to test substances that would increase the work capacity of soldiers at the front during World War II. Upon graduation, Dr. Brekhman continued his research, applying scientific method to the study of plants, investigating their biological activity, unraveling their genetic codes, and elucidating their adaptogenic properties. He studied Panax ginseng from the orient and set out to find a cheaper and a more readily available substitute for this traditional Chinese herb. He soon discovered Siberian ginseng and found that it was not only readily available but also surpassed Panax ginseng in potency. This event ignited Dr. Brekhman's interest in discovering plants that possessed adaptogenic properties. As his work progressed and word of his amazing discoveries reached Soviet authorities, he was commissioned by the Russian government to further his studies for more "applicable" purposes.

Dr. Brekhman's formulas, a product of his extensive work with adaptogenic plants, were used by the Russian cosmonauts to protect against the stresses of space flight, including weightlessness and inactivity. Performance artists, master chess players, and top ranking Soviet officials all used Brekhman's formulas to excel in their fields. During the 1970s and 1980s, Dr. Brekhman led a team of Russian sports scientists studying the use of natural substances for enhancing performance and strength as a substitute for anabolic steroids. Once again, they focused their attention on adaptogens. Their research and formulas led to breakthroughs in performance and endurance that placed Soviet athletes first among their competition. For 45 years this visionary looked to nature, "the greatest laboratory on earth," as he once said, and thus, he found Rhodiola rosea.

Rhodiola rosea: Nature's Panacea in a Plant

Rhodiola rosea, also known as "arctic root" or "golden root," is a member of the family Crassulaceae, plants indigenous to the polar arctic regions of eastern Siberia, growing at altitudes of 11,000 to 18,000 feet above sea level. Its height reaches almost two and a half feet. Its yellow flowers smell similar to attar of roses, thus the name "rosea."

Historically, only members of extended families knew where this precious plant grew, and the means to prepare it—knowledge passed on from generation to generation. In Siberia it is said, "people who drink Rhodiola rosea tea will live more than 100 years." For many centuries, Chinese emperors commissioned special expeditions to eastern Siberia and Altai to discover where "golden root" grew and to bring it back to China for the treatment of disease. So valued was this commodity that, for many years, Rhodiola rosea was illegally shipped across the Russian border to China. No doubt those caught suffered severe penalties. Rhodiola rosea was also one of the most popular medicinal herbs in middle Asia. In these countries, a tea made from the plant is administered during the cold and wet Asian winters to prevent sickness. Mongolian doctors also prescribed Rhodiola rosea extract for the treatment of tuberculosis and cancer.

Initially, with most research devoted to Siberian ginseng, research on Rhodiola rosea was very limited. Combined with the fact that Rhodiola rosea was a scarce commodity, its usefulness seemed nearly impractical. This was about to change, however, when scientists from the Tomsk State University found places where Rhodiola rosea still grew wild at elevations 5000 to 9000 feet above sea level in the Siberian mountains, making the plant at least more available for further research. And what the researchers found was amazing. Taken with Rhodiola rosea's legendary history of beneficial effects, it is easy to understand why this powerful adaptogenic plant became one of Russia's best-kept secrets.

Fortunately, by the early 1990s, information on the extraordinary health benefits of Rhodiola rosea were released to the world. More recent research and its results have dramatically increased the interest in this miraculous species of plant. Pharmacological study of a preparation of Rhodiola rosea, for example, has shown it to be such powerful medicine that clinical trials were recommended. Several of these trials, all double-blind and placebo controlled, provided even stronger evidence that Rhodiola rosea possessed high biological activity with **no detectable levels of toxicity.** Rhodiola rosea is not just another adaptogen from Russia. Like Siberian ginseng, Rhodiola rosea possesses several unique properties that set it apart from other adaptogens.

Rhodiola 101

Different Rhodiola species have been found not only in the former Soviet Union but also in Europe and the Caucasian Mountains of Georgian Republic (Table 2.2). Russian scientists have identified nearly 200 species, 14 of which have undergone intensive investigation. The chemical composition and pharmacological activity of Rhodiola is strongly a species-dependent phenomenon. The plant is a hodgepodge of phytochemicals, including phenylpropanoids, proanthocyanidins, and flavonoids (see Figures 2.1 to 2.13). The most important chemical molecules that were scien-

Table 2.2 The Rhodiola Family

Rhodiola Family
Rhodiola rosea
Rhodiola quadfida
Rhodiola gelida
Rhodiola heterodonta
Rhodiola sacchalinensis
Rhodiola pinnatifida
Rhodiola kirilowii
Rhodiola crenulata
Rhodiola coccinea
Rhodiola alterna
Rhodiola brevipetiolata
Rhodiola wolongensis
Rhodiola fastigita
Rhodiola ellipticum

tifically and clinically proven to be very active are the phenylpropanoids, rosavin (the most active), rosin, rosarin, rhodiolin, salidroside, and its aglycon, p–tyrosol. What sets Rhodiola rosea apart from other species in this family? According to researchers, only Rhodiola rosea contains rosavin and its related phytochemicals, rosin and rosarin. So out of all the different species, Rhodiola rosea is the most biologically active.

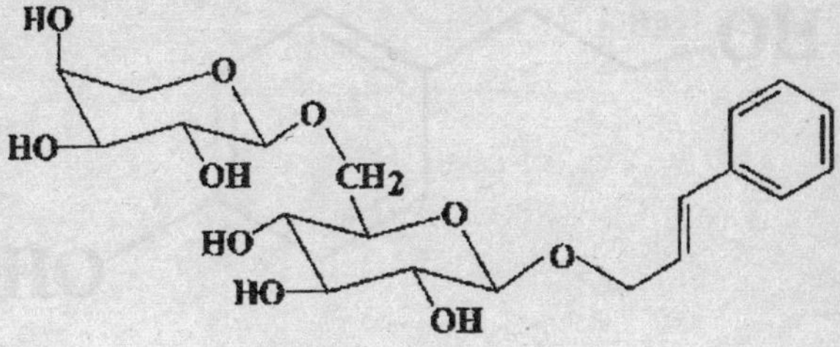

Figure 2.1 Rosavin

It is important to understand that if one is seeking an effective Rhodiola rosea extract, it must be standardized for the important actives, rosavin and salidroside. It must contain rosavin because the presence of salidroside alone is not specific to Rhodiola rosea at all! Many plants within the Rhodiola genus contain salidroside and other plants, including White Willow *(Salix)* and the evergreen medicinal plant Rhododendron, also contain salidroside. Therefore, it is absolutely clear that the use of salidroside without rosavin, for the identification and standardization of Rhodiola rosea, is inaccurate and will not ensure its promised effectiveness.

Thus as we have noted, while other species of Rhodiola do possess some pharmacological properties, only Rhodiola rosea has been used for more than 30 years,

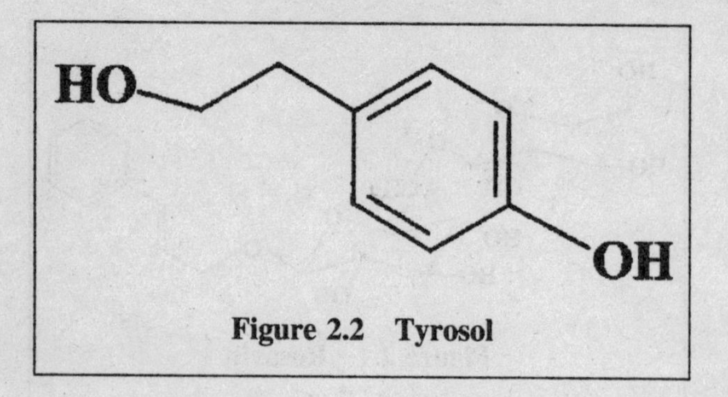

Figure 2.2 Tyrosol

in both animal and human studies, and has proven to be safe. This cannot be said for other Rhodiola species.

What is the connection, then, between Rhodiola rosea and disease? We know that the body's ability to resist stress is defined by its ability to counteract the excessive demands placed upon it. As a majority of illnesses have their roots in stress, if we could ameliorate the effects of stress, we could also theoretically at least prevent disease. During the more than 30 years Rhodiola rosea has been studied a sizeable amount of evidence has built up suggesting that it can prevent disease via its adaptogenic properties. In the following chapters you will begin to see how stress is intimately tied to disease and illness, and how Rhodiola rosea, the only species in its family, can thwart stress' malignant effects.

Recommended Dose

Standardized Rhodiola rosea
(standardized for rosavin and salidroside):
200–300mg daily with meals

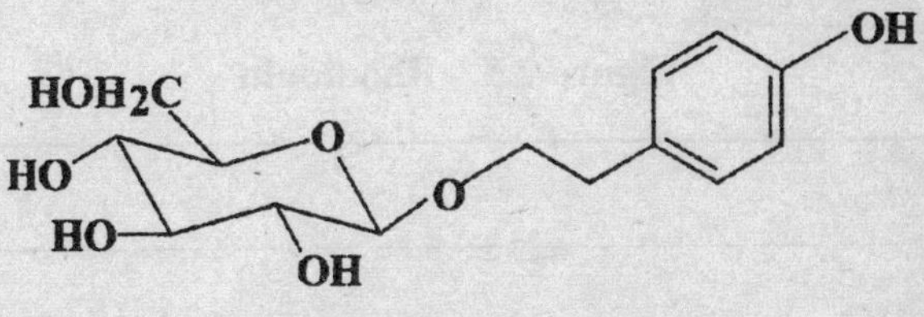

Figure 2.3 Salidroside

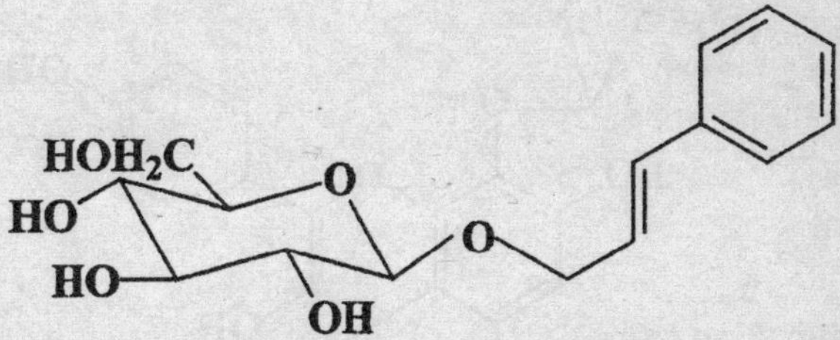

Figure 2.4 Rosin

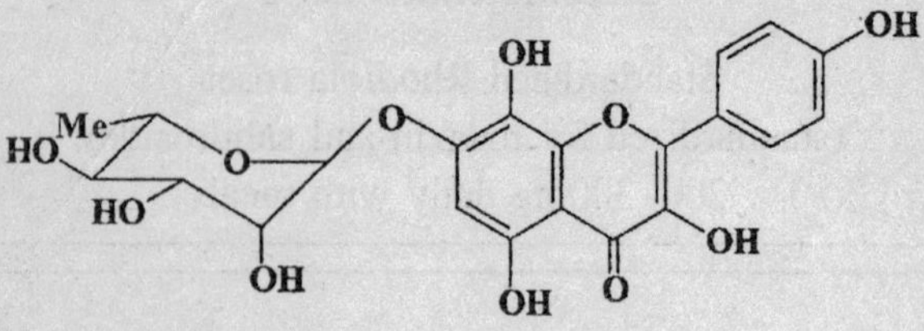

Figure 2.5 Rhodionin

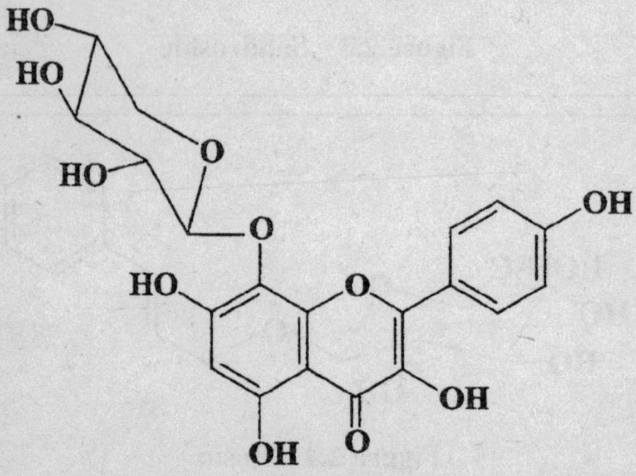

Figure 2.6 Rhodalin

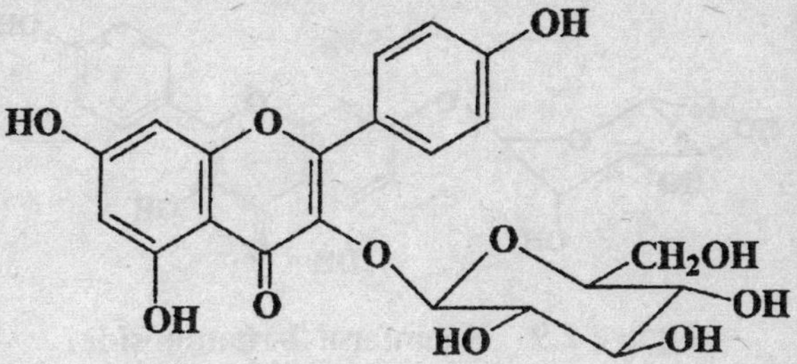

Figure 2.7 Astragalin

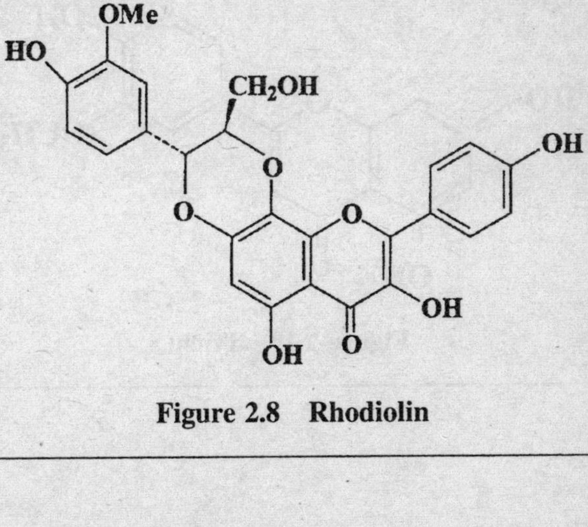

Figure 2.8 Rhodiolin

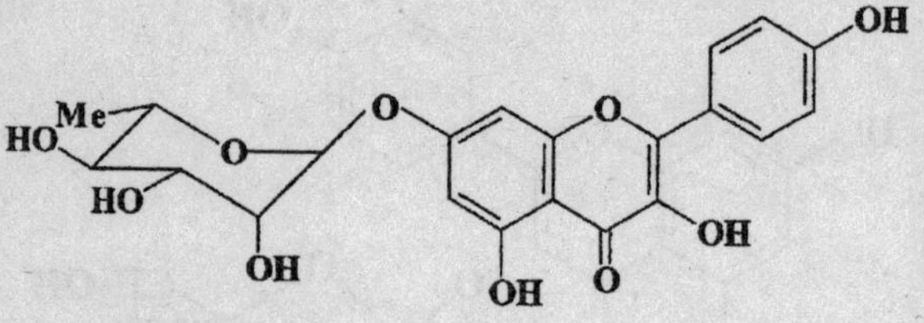

Figure 2.9 Kaemferol 7-rhamnoside

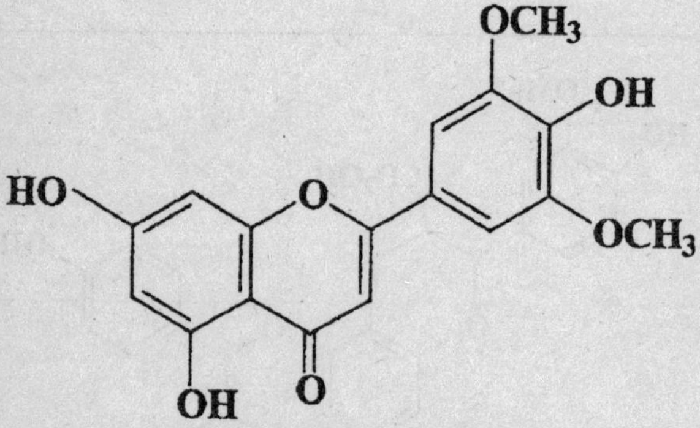

Figure 2.10 Tricin

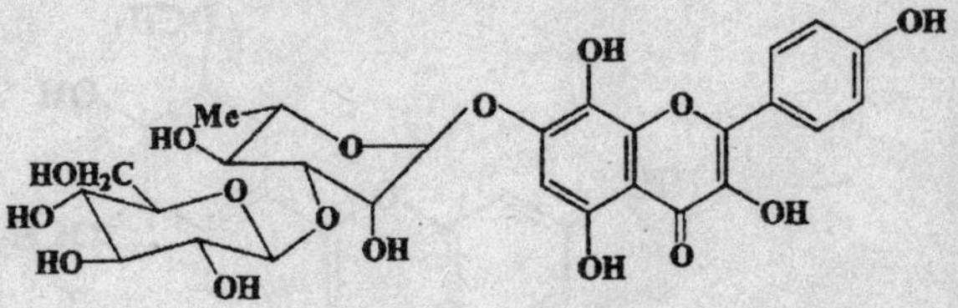

Figure 2.11 Rhodiosin

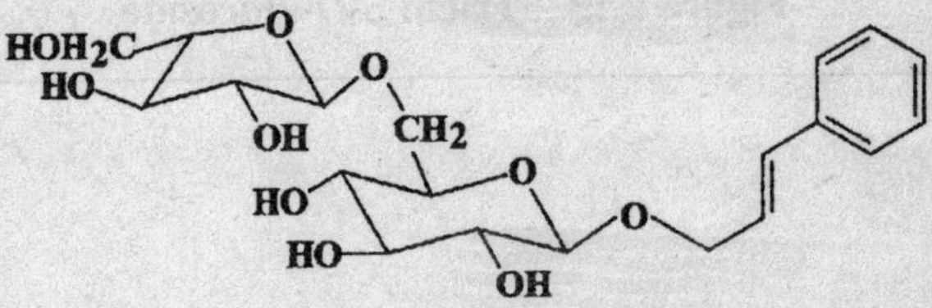

Figure 2.12 Rosarin

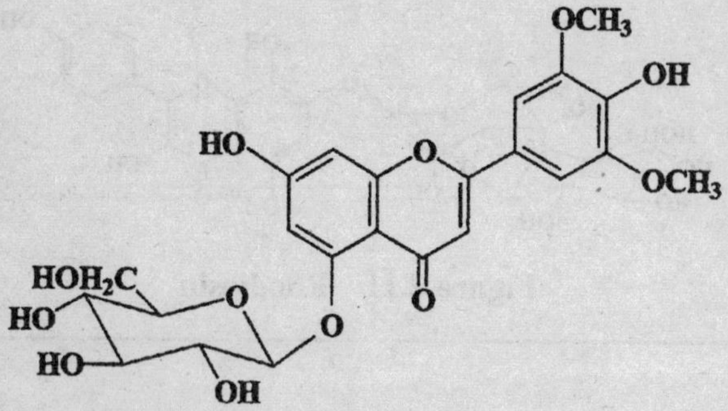

Figure 2.13 Tricin 5-*O*-glucoside

CHAPTER 3

Rhodiola rosea and Depression

Depression: A Positive Note Without Prozac?

Depression is a complex interplay of both physiological and psychological processes that ultimately culminate in feelings of sadness, indifference, and irritability. Normal sleep patterns are disrupted and the victim's appetite and weight may vary considerably. They feel encumbered with fatigue and find it difficult to think clearly and concentrate. Often, feelings of shame or guilt and a preoccupation with death or dying occupy their thoughts. Approximately 15 percent of the general population suffers from major depressive episodes with the incidence increasing with age. Depression is also a disproportionate disease, affecting women twice as much as men, regardless of age.

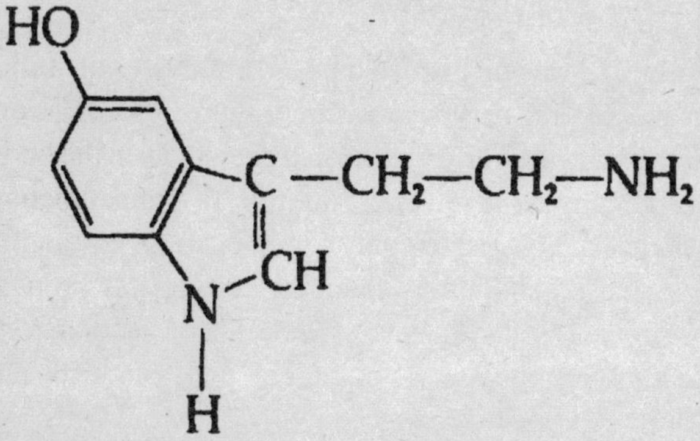

Figure 3.1 Serotonin is a chemical found naturally throughout the body that plays a critical role in regulating brain function.

As for the rest of us, bouts of occasional depression are normal and precipitate from something as superficial as a rainy day to the tragedy of losing a loved one. Of course when the depression becomes persistent rather than episodic, therapy is an alternative. Evidence also suggests that Rhodiola rosea may help those people, buried by feelings of depression, climb out of their psychological hole. How does Rhodiola rosea work to restore mental health? Before I reveal Rhodiola rosea's beneficial properties, it's important to understand a little about neurology.

Serotonin: A "Jack of all Trades"

Serotonin was first isolated in 1948 and later identified in the central nervous system (Figure 3.1). It is one of the most actively investigated chemicals in the body, specifically as it relates to its role in brain function. The brain, however, is only a small part of serotonin's effect. This ubiquitous chemical participates in many processes, including smooth muscle contraction, temperature regulation, appetite, pain perception, behavior, blood pressure, and respiration. Serotonin, because of its ability to constrict blood vessels, has been suggested as a possible treatment for migraine headaches, which occur when blood vessels in the brain dilate. The largest pool of serotonin is seen in the gastrointestinal tract where it may regulate gastric motility, the ability of the digestive organs to move substances through them. Although the amount of serotonin in the brain is comparatively small (one to two percent), when compared to other parts of the body its importance in brain function cannot be underestimated.

Within the brain lies extensive collections of serotonin-containing neurons in an area called the raphe nuclei—and it is here where serotonin is active. Unfortunately, however, serotonin is unable to cross the blood–brain barrier, a semipermeable membrane that regulates the passage of certain substances into the brain. Its biosynthesis, therefore, must begin in the brain itself. Enter the essential amino acid, tryptophan, serotonin's raw material. Tryptophan can cross the blood–brain barrier and, within the brain, it is converted to 5–hydroxytryptophan (5–HTP) by the enzyme tryptophan hydroxylase. The final step involves the conversion of 5–HTP to 5–hydroxytryptamine (5–HT), otherwise known as serotonin.

Throughout the body a system of checks and balances works to keep us healthy. Nowhere is this more evident than in the control of serotonin production in the brain. Two powerful enzymes, monoamine oxidase and aldehyde dehydrogenase, act to limit the production of serotonin. Without them, too much serotonin would be produced, which is just as bad as too little serotonin. Like the body, then, brain function is dependent on maintaining its proper balance, here, between serotonin and the enzymes that inactivate it. When this balance is altered, so is health.

Slight disturbances in serotonin balance lead to substantial deviations in personality. Anxiety, obsessive-compulsive disorder, schizophrenia and, of course, depression have all been associated with reduced levels of serotonin. Serotonin was first implicated in the etiology of depression from evidence of drugs that precipitated and relieved depressive symptoms. These drugs were effective in treating depression effectively by increasing levels of serotonin in the brain. It is this neurotransmitter that pharmaceutical companies have sought to correct in people suffering from depression. Anyone ever heard of Prozac?

Stress and Depression: Burning the "Psychological Candle" at Both Ends

The research supporting stress' role in depression is accumulating. Various studies demonstrated that significantly higher emotional stress resulted in greater depressive episodes and higher tension, anxiety, anger, hostility, confusion, and fatigue. This kind of reaction occurs more frequently in older rather than younger adults. For example, college students who advance from basic science training to more clinical training experience a concomitant increase in stress and depressed mood. Observations of Alzheimer's disease caregivers who experience this stressful life event are prone to depression and poorer health than individuals with less stress. It is apparent that emotional and psychological stresses take their toll and lead to feelings of depression, anxiety, and even anger. The resulting alterations in serotonin metabolism attest to stress' profound effect in the brain.

Transmission of serotonin in certain regions of brain cells called the raphe nucleus is thought to be under the control of certain receptors known as $5\text{–}HT_{1A}$. These serotonin receptors play a key role in the regulation of electrical and metabolic activity of serotonin-activated neurons in the raphe nucleus. These same neurons, however, contain receptors for glucocorticoids, the hormones released into the body during stress. Glucocorticoids may be involved in the modulation of serotonin by desensitizing 5–HT receptors and thus attenuating serotonin's effects. In fact, research has suggested this same concept and has demonstrated that stress can reduce the electrophysiological activity of serotonin-activated neurons in the raphe nucleus.

Additional evidence supporting stress as an antagonist to serotonin comes from blood platelets, small oval disks found in the circulatory system, which play an important role in blood coagulation and clotting. Blood platelets also contain receptors on their surface that are similar to serotonin receptors found in the brain and, therefore, are a convenient way to measure serotonin metabolism during stressful episodes. Researchers have taken advantage of the similarities and investigated the effects of post-traumatic stress disorder (PTSD) on serotonin. Exposure to extreme trauma and a real or perceived threat to one's life may trigger a PTSD response. The subject develops significant anxiety and mood alterations similar to depression.

Investigators used paroxetine, a chemical similar to serotonin in that it binds readily to serotonin receptors. When they examined individuals suffering from post-traumatic stress disorder, they found that the amount of paroxetine bound to serotonin receptors decreased. What is more astonishing here is that, upon closer observation, researchers discovered that the number of binding sites on the platelet surface decreased as well! So not only did stress decrease paroxetine's ability to bind to the same receptors that serotonin binds to, but it also decreased the number of functional binding sites. This same phenomenon has been seen in suicide victims with a history of depression.

Taken collectively, alteration in sensitivity to serotonin and a reduction in serotonin's ability to bind nerve cells may explain why stress induces depressive episodes, but what about the neurotransmitter itself? Can stress decrease serotonin synthesis? In a study using animal models exposed to acute and chronic forms of stress, within 18 hours of acute stress, a twofold *decrease* of serotonin levels was seen in the brain cortex. Evidence is also mounting that serotonin itself may play a role in stress protection. The serotoninergic system of the brain participates in the formation of the stress reaction and plays a major role in the mechanism of adaptation to new environmental conditions. In a stressful situation, however, the amount of serotonin in the brain decreases. In other words, serotonin may be involved in Dr. Selye's "general adaptation syndrome." During the "resistance phase," serotonin may heighten our ability to resist stress. As the reserves diminish, however, so does our ability to combat stress, resulting in "exhaustion." Today, there are many magazine articles and books written about depression. Russian scientists have found in Rhodiola rosea a powerful weapon for combating this scourge of modern life.

Rhodiola Rosea: Soviet St. John's Wort?

As we noted previously, and before Rhodiola Rosea was released to the world, clinical studies on Rhodiola rosea were performed only at leading Soviet universities and medical academies, with their results kept secret for decades. Because Soviet authorities never controlled the science behind projects related to Siberian ginseng projects, the "closed" science on Rhodiola rosea did provoke many speculations. However, we now understand that the secrecy surrounding research with Rhodiola rosea was also based upon scientific considerations. Quite simply, Rhodiola rosea possesses extraordinary medicinal properties. As an adaptogen, researchers concluded that Rhodiola rosea is much more powerful than other adaptogens, including Panax ginseng, Siberian ginseng, schizandra, and aralia. Rhodiola rosea's powerful antidepressive effects are a testament to its potent adaptogenic properties.

A positive therapeutic effect of Rhodiola rosea was shown in patients with pronounced depressive states of varied origins. One hundred twenty-eight individuals, ages 17 to 55 years, were observed. After the administration of the Rhodiola rosea preparation, a substantial decrease or complete disappearance of the clinical manifestations of depression was noted in 65 percent of the patients. The subjective improvement of the patient's condition was confirmed by psychological testing, as well as increased work productivity.

In another experiment, patients suffering from paranoid experiences or profound emotional alterations took 100 milligrams of Rhodiola rosea twice a day for one to four months. Symptoms, including general weakness, increased fragility, daytime sleepiness and disturbances in nocturnal sleep, either decreased or disappeared altogether. In those patients with deep depressive manifestations, improvements were noted almost across the board. They became more sociable, and more active, and their motivational levels increased. These clinical studies demonstrate that Rhodiola rosea extract significantly decreases and/or eliminates depressive symptomatology. How, then, does Rhodiola rosea accomplish a feat that was once thought to be the sole privilege of pharmaceutical drugs?

The Rhodiola and Serotonin Connection

Remember: Depression is a consequence of insufficient serotonin levels. In response, scientists have found that extracts of Rhodiola rosea, namely rosavin and salidroside, enhance the transport of the serotonin precursors, tryptophan, and 5–hydroxytryptophan, into the brain. Initial evidence supporting this hypothesis came from animal studies demonstrating 5–HTP induced hyperkinesis, a condition characterized by abnormally increased motor function and convulsive shaking of the head due to excessive serotonin levels

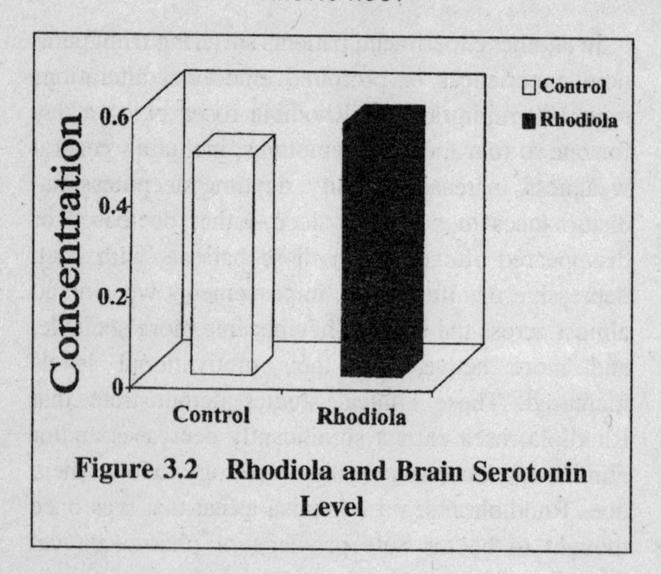

Figure 3.2 Rhodiola and Brain Serotonin Level

in the brain. In effect, researchers can cause a hyperkinetic reaction by administering excessive levels of 5–HTP, which are quickly absorbed by the brain and converted to serotonin. Serotonin levels rise and result in hyperkinesis.

Rhodiola rosea, when given in combination with 5–HTP, intensified 5–HTP's hyperkinetic effect. This means that Rhodiola rosea enhances the uptake of serotonin precursors into the brain and greater availability correlates to greater serotonin synthesis and, you guessed it, increased serotonin levels (Figure 3.2). Additionally, research points to Rhodiola rosea playing a more important role in preserving serotonin rather than increasing its biosynthesis. Serotonin and other amines normally inactivated by the enzyme catechol-O-methyl transferase (COMT) are spared due to Rhodiola rosea's ability to inhibit the activity of these powerful enzymes. Professors A.S. Saratikov and T.F. Marina, prominent Soviet scientists, have shown that Rhodiola rosea can increase serotonin levels by 30 percent and decrease COMT activity by 60 percent!

Earlier in this chapter we discussed serotonin's ability to help the body adapt to stress and that decreases in serotonin results from various prolonged stresses. Rhodiola rosea's ability to help the body adapt to stress may lie in its ability to enhance serotonin levels. In other words, it is not Rhodiola rosea that facilitates adaptation, it is serotonin, supported by Rhodiola rosea that causes a change. Thus, Rhodiola rosea conforms to the prerequisite for adaptogens, "nonspecific" and "normalizing." Rhodiola rosea's proven effectiveness for depression has led Russian scientists to use it in combination with antidepressants. Patient's general activity, including levels of intellectual and physical productivity, increased while length of stay in the hospital and side effects associated with tricyclic antidepressants decreased. Rhodiola rosea is a safe and effective adjunct to conventional antidepressant therapy. For those of us who suffer from the occasional "blue Monday," Rhodiola rosea is an effective and welcome supplement to boost our spirits naturally.

Recommended Daily Antidepressant Formula	
Standardized Rhodiola rosea	200 mg
Standardized St. John's Wort	200 mg
DHA (docosahexaneoic acid)	300 mg
PS (phosphatidylserine)	300 mg
Inositol	3 grams
SAM (s–adenosyl methionine)	200 mg
Chromium (glycinate)	200 mcg
General Multiple Vitamin & Mineral Formula—as per label directions	

CHAPTER 4

Rhodiola rosea and the Heart

The Heart

Perhaps the most important muscle in the body is the heart. It's a marvelous little pump that beats tirelessly and inconspicuously every day of every month of every year. It is also one of the most exploited. We take it for granted that the heart will beat reliably and consistently every day, even though we abuse it with poor or inadequate diet and lack of exercise. Like an overworked and underpaid employee, the heart has its limitations, and, after repeated exposure to adverse conditions, it simply quits. An unhealthy lifestyle with generous amounts of stress is the recipe for disaster, and it's a recipe we prepare all too often. Before we can understand how stress affects the heart though, we must understand how the heart works as a pump.

Heart Physiology: A Cursory Review

Think of the heart as a two-story house with two rooms on top and two on the bottom. The second floor rooms are the atriums of the heart that collect and move the blood from circulation to the lower level of the house, the ventricles. The ventricles are the largest rooms in the house, and they have to be because it is their job to eject the blood out of the heart and back into circulation. In order for the heart to function properly and move blood efficiently throughout the body, it must contract in a controlled and rhythmic fashion. Unlike other muscles in the body that require a stimulus from the central nervous system, however, the cardiac muscle is self-excitable or "myogenic." It can contract without any signals from the brain. This presents a problem. Because the heart is not regulated by the brain, specialized, highly excitable, cells within the heart, called "pacemaker cells" must exist. If these pacemaker cells were absent, the heart would soon become only a quivering mound of muscle. These cells set the rhythm for the entire heart and form a conduction system by which the impulse can move through the entire heart in a controlled and coordinated manner.

This conduction system, as it is called, consists of specialized areas called the sinoatrial node (SA), atrioventricular node (AV), bundle of His, and the Purkinje fibers. Normally, excitation begins in the sinoatrial node, located in the right atrium, and from there the impulse moves to the atrioventricular node, bundle of His, and finally the Purkinje fibers. When the impulse reaches the AV node, there is a pause in the transference of the impulse to the rest of the conduction system and thus a pause in the contraction of the heart between the "first and second floors." In essence, then, the four chambers of the heart—the two atriums and the two ventricles—are "timed" between atrial and ventricular activity. In other words, the heart actually beats twice. The first contraction is the atriums (via excitation of the SA node) injecting blood into the ventricles, with the second contraction via the ventricles (through excitation of the AV node, bundle of His, and Purkinje fibers), which finally eject blood out of the heart and into the rest of the body.

Without this conduction system, the heart would beat out of control. More importantly, without calcium, sodium, and potassium the conduction system would not work at all—for these same minerals are needed to "excite" the cardiac cells. Normally, the amount of sodium and calcium outside of the cells is high, relative to the amount within the cell. The opposite is true for potassium. In order for the cardiac cell to contract, there must be an influx of sodium and calcium into the cell. It does this by activating specialized structures in the cell membrane called "sodium and calcium" channels. These channels are analogous to the front door of the house, opening to allow sodium and calcium to enter the cell. Once these minerals enter the cell, physiological events take place to cause cardiac cells to contract. This entire process is known as "depolarization." The heart contracts when the multitude of cells that make up the muscle fibers contract instantaneously.

Contraction, however, must end in order for the heart to refill with blood and begin another contraction cycle. At this point, potassium is key. During recovery from contraction "potassium channels" within the cell membrane open, allowing potassium to exit the cell while at the same time sodium and calcium channels are closing. As more potassium exits, the cardiac cell "relaxes," and this relaxation is subsequently transferred to the entire heart. Scientists have termed this phenomenon "repolarization."

Left to its own accord this process would continue indefinitely and regularly. Ignorantly, the heart would beat without any regard for us. But there are times when the heart rate must increase to compensate for demands placed on the body. Demands, such as physical exercise or the "fight or flight" response, necessitate increased cardiac output. In this regard, the responsibility of increased cardiac performance falls to the autonomic nervous system and the adrenal glands.

Sympathetic Nervous System (SNS) and Adrenal Glands: Mind (and Glands) over Muscle

The nervous system's control of heart rate stems from the cardiovascular center in the medulla of the brain. From there a signal propagates along sympathetic nerve fibers which innervate with the SA and AV nodes of the heart. The SNS unconsciously and quickly "jump-starts" the heart rate and enhances the heart's ability to contract. It does this by releasing norepinephrine locally and increasing calcium entry in the cardiac cell. Like the SNS, the catecholamines, epinephrine and norepinephrine, products of the adrenal glands, accelerate heart rate and increase contractility of heart muscle during stress. The adrenal glands support the activity of the SNS and prolong the heightened cardiac response to stress.

So, the same systems involved in the stress response (sympathetic nervous system and the adrenal glands) are intimately connected to heart function. Again, in terms of evolution, these regulatory devices were important when defense, either by fighting or running, becomes imperative. Unfortunately, those same mechanisms that protected us from danger in the past are killing us today. The only difference between then and now is how much and how long the stress lasts. In modern society, chronic exposure to emotional and psychological stress leads to a constant stimulation of the heart by the stress response systems. Eventually, the heart reaches a breaking point manifesting itself as the number one killer of American people: heart disease.

Stress and the Heart

Approximately 22.3 million Americans will be diagnosed with heart disease this year, with 700,000 losing their lives because of it. Heart disease is the number one cause of death in the United States. Among the risk factors associated with heart disease (Table 4.1), stress has reared its ugly head and, in fact, may play a greater role contributing to the statistics than previously thought.

The American Heart Association correlates anxiety, depression, emotional drain, and conflict with increased incidence of angina pectoris, an acute pain in the chest resulting from a decreased blood supply to the heart. In fact, using 132 patients with coronary artery disease, scientists found that emotional stress can trigger a decrease in the blood supply to the heart and that high levels of mental stress more than doubles the risk of ischemia (reduced blood supply to the heart). What does this say about the general population, those of us who do not (yet) show signs of heart disease? The fact that stress affects normal heart function may be more inconspicuous and insidious in healthy hearts than in diseased hearts, which trigger a pain response when stressed. ‘‘Out of sight, out of mind’’ is our

Table 4.1 Risk Factors for Heart Disease

- High blood cholesterol
- High blood pressure
- Cigarette smoking
- Obesity
- Lack of regular exercise
- Diabetes mellitus
- Genetic predisposition
- Male gender
- Stress

motto as aggravation, worry, anger, and irritability cause over-stimulation of the sympathetic nervous system and adrenal glands. It is only when pain or a heart attack occurs that we think about what we could have done differently. The connection between stress and heart disease simply cannot be discounted.

Researchers reporting in the *American Journal of Medicine* have demonstrated increased risk of cardiovascular disease among patients being treated for rheumatoid arthritis. A distinguishing characteristic of this population was that the therapy entailed the use of corticosteroids, the same chemicals the body produces during stress. Every day we are subject to constant emotional stress from every angle. Although the evidence associating heart disease with stress is accumulating, science still speculates as to how stress affects the heart.

Stress: Mechanism of Morbidity

Stress may play an important role influencing other factors correlated to heart disease, such as cholesterol, obesity, diabetes, and hypertension. Catecholamines induce the release of lipids and glucose into the bloodstream, raising cholesterol levels and exacerbating diabetes. The association between stress and hypertension may be more pertinent than previously thought and can be especially problematic among those suffering from hypertension. In an article published in the *Journal of Nervous and Mental Disease,* investigators reviewed 48 studies examining the relationship between blood pressure and psychosocial variables. They found that a strong association between hypertension and the psychosocial factors of anger, hostility, interpersonal anxiety, and the use of inhibiting defense mechanisms (i.e., denial and repression) existed. These emotional "cannonballs" are the product of challenges we undertake every day *and* our inability to express these emotions because of societal repression against them. Certainly, such emotions contribute to breaking down our defenses against stress.

More importantly, stress may prove to be more of

a potent risk factor, independent of other risk factors. The outpouring of epinephrine, norepinephrine, and cortisol may have a more direct effect on the heart, damaging the very tissue itself and disrupting rhythmic contraction. Researchers have shown that animals infused with catecholamines almost immediately develop over-contracted cardiac muscle fibers, known as ''contraction band lesions.'' These lesions are the result of heart muscle contracting so severely that the actual fibers rupture, resulting in a microscopic band of dead cells. As a result, not only does this section of heart muscle become dysfunctional, it can also disrupt the natural and coordinated conduction of the impulse that travels through the heart muscle itself. With a disrupted conduction system the heart beats out of sequence, a condition known as arrhythmia. The corticosteroids released during the stress response are also potassium-wasting; that is, they increase potassium excretion from the body. As a result, potassium, the mineral needed to relax cardiac muscle, may be substantially lost during stressful situations and may further irritate arrhythmic conditions.

Contraction band lesions, cardiac arrhythmias, and stress may explain why heart attacks are so prevalent in America: the greater the levels of stress hormones, the greater the amount of contraction band lesions; the greater the contraction band lesions, the greater the likelihood of arrhythmias; the greater the likelihood of arrhythmia, the greater the likelihood of sudden cardiac death (abrupt and unexpected heart failure). Contraction band lesions are seen in 86 percent of sudden cardiac death victims. Do we see a pattern here? High levels of the stress hormones may precipitate a heart attack because of their ability to alter the normal conduction of heart impulses. A very complex relation indeed, but then again, so is Rhodiola rosea's cardio-protective properties.

Rhodiola rosea: Getting to the Heart of the Problem

There is no question that Rhodiola rosea prevents cardiac damage by decreasing the amount of catecholamines and corticosteroids released during the stress response and subsequently decreasing the ''adrenaline burn'' on the heart. Rhodiola rosea's normalizing effect on the adrenal glands may also normalize cholesterol, blood sugar, potassium levels, and blood pressure thereby decreasing risk factors for heart disease. Isolates from Rhodiola rosea were shown to decrease serum levels of cholesterol and triglycerides in animal models. According to these researchers, the therapeutic effect was associated with both hypolipidemic (lipid lowering) activity and ability to enhance the resistance of the vascular wall to cholesterol infiltration. The latter is purported to play a significant role in heart disease. Rhodiola's ability to alter the risk factors for heart disease is significant but doesn't stop there.

Rhodiola rosea decreases the amount of cyclic–AMP (c–AMP) released into cardiac cells. Cyclic–AMP is a distant cousin of ATP (adenosine triphosphate), the body's primary energy molecule. When activated, c–AMP acts as a "second messenger" or a liaison between the outer and inner environments of the cell. One of its roles in the heart is to stimulate the release of more calcium into the heart cell and, thus, promote greater potential for the muscle to contract. Thus, Rhodiola rosea may protect the heart by maintaining normal c–AMP levels during stressful situations, and prevent a heightened state of cardiac contraction.

Perhaps the most astonishing find is Rhodiola rosea's anti-arrhythmic effect through the opioids. You may be familiar with the term "opiates," drugs such as morphine used in the medical industry to relieve pain. Opioids are a class of compounds, similar in structure and function to opiates, that our bodies produce to reduce the sensation of pain. The endorphins, enkephalins, and dynorphins, as they are classified, are essential for pain regulation. Did you ever feel numb after breaking an arm or injuring some other part of your body? That's the opioids in your body kicking in. Recent evidence points to the opioids participating in cardio-protection, and Rhodiola rosea may enhance these "pain killer/heart helper" chemicals.

Initial evidence of Rhodiola rosea modulating the opioid system came from animals experiencing epinephrine-induced arrhythmias. When Rhodiola rosea was administered, the animals experienced a significant resistance to arrhythmias. But when injected with naloxone, a drug that antagonizes opioid effectiveness, Rhodiola rosea's protective effects were negated. Even though we do not fully understand Rhodiola rosea's cardio-protective effects, those effects are either the result of a direct interaction of the herb with opioid receptors or indirectly through enhanced opioid synthesis.

The role opioids play in protecting the heart against arrhythmia and even ischemic insult is new and exciting. Interactions between opioids, opioid receptors, and Rhodiola rosea are complex and require further investigation to fully understand the interplay between them. Opioids may be involved in ischemic preconditioning, a process by which the heart becomes increasingly resistant to cardiac tissue damage due to low oxygen and blood supply to the heart. Rhodiola rosea has shown it can play an effective role in protecting the tissues of the heart, which enables this vital organ to function normally.

Recommended Daily Heart Protective Formula

Standardized Rhodiola rosea	200 mg
Vitamin E (tocopherols)	400 IU
L–Carnitine	500 mg
Coenzyme Q-10	100 mg
Soy Isoflavone Concentrate	100 mg
Magnesium (glycinate)	400 mg
Taurine	500 mg
Grape Seed Extract	60 mg
Standardized Hawthorne Berry	150 mg
Pantethine	200 mg
Standardized Garlic	200 mg

General Multiple Vitamin/Mineral Supplement

CHAPTER 5

Rhodiola rosea and Immunity

It was a moonless night. The air was warm, but the sounds of war raged through my land. Constantly the invaders are at my heels, attacking my beautiful castle day after day. No treaty will keep them off my borders; no truce will turn them away. Although my forces are strong and brave, sometimes I wonder how we manage to beat them back every time. Just yesterday the horrid beasts made it through our first defense: an acrid moat surrounding the castle. Then the tar bogs failed to even slow them down, so I sent out my best scouts. Fierce hulking men, they are trained to attack any invader who threatens our way of life. Even at the gates of death these brave souls will destroy their enemy, placing the beast's helmet on a spear for all to see. Seeing the enemy forces growing, I signaled for my herald to open the drawbridge to let my soldiers out in numbers. They swung into action, surrounding the enemy on all sides. Archers fired arrows into the air like a deadly rain, and my buglers sounded out a triumphant note, calling more of my courageous soldiers into the fray. Just as I thought the battle was over, one of my palace guardsmen brought me a soldier who he had found to be engaged in traitorous activity. The deceit never ends, but I know now that the next time we are attacked, I will be better prepared to ward off the invaders, and the children of these brave soldiers will be trained at an early age to defeat these monsters.

The Invaders

Although the above may read like a passage in a medieval fantasy novel, this type of battle goes on inside our body every moment of our lives. Just replace the "invaders" with some nasty bacteria or viruses, the soldiers with our immune system, and the castle with our cells, and the picture becomes clear. The "battle scene" metaphor also depicts how crucial our immune system is to our lives. Simply put, we would die without it, and yet so many influences, such as daily stress, can damage our immune system and render it useless. Before we investigate the effect of stress on the immune system and the connection between our hero—Rhodiola rosea—and stress, it will be helpful to delve into the inner workings of our wonderful immune system to see what it's all about.

The First Line of Defense: Skin and Mucous

In the example above, the invaders needed to wade through an ''acrid moat'' and ''tar pits'' to gain access to the castle. In real life, all forms of invading microorganisms must first get through our largest organ (the skin) to pose any threat. In itself, the skin presents a formidable mechanical barrier. Due to our natural oils and perspiration, it also presents a chemical barrier: It is too acidic for most microorganisms to set up camp on. If any pathogens are lucky enough to circumvent the skin and find a way into the body, it is likely that mucous secretions will immobilize them. A good example of this defense system is in the respiratory tract, lined with tiny hairs that keep mucous secretions and trapped bacteria moving away from the lungs and out of the body. In light of this information, it is easy to see how reactions like coughing and sneezing are really the body's way of expelling harmful microorganisms and normally should not be suppressed.

Inflammation and the Phagocytes: Opening the Drawbridge

When the skin is punctured or damaged in some way, the local tissue becomes swollen and red. This reaction is yet another of the body's immune defenses called the "inflammatory response." Inflammation causes capillaries to leak and dilate, allowing immune cells to migrate out of the blood vessels to the damaged tissue. In our metaphor, the herald who opened the drawbridge to let out more soldiers played the part of a compound called "histamine," which further increases the leakiness of capillaries. Those suffering from allergies are well acquainted with the effects of histamine: runny nose, teary eyes, and itchiness. Although it is critical for the immune response, it can present a problem when released in excessive amounts.

The immune cells that leak out of the capillaries and into surrounding tissue are called "phagocytes" (in our metaphor, the scouts). Basically, there are two types of phagocytes: neutrophils and macrophages. Neutrophils are usually the first to arrive on the scene, scavenging and engulfing bacteria and viruses alike. Macrophages not only engulf pathogens, but they also present a part of it on their own cell membrane called an "antigen" (the helmet in the metaphor). Other cells of the immune system, called "Helper T cells," recognize and interact with these antigens and stimulate the macrophage to release interleukin 1, a chemical that increases T cell proliferation. Interleukin 1 also induces helper T cells to release Interleukin 2, which causes a subsequent rise in the number of another type of T cell, called "cytotoxic T cells." Like the archers above, cytotoxic T cells destroy pathogens directly by punching holes in their cell membrane and causing them to break apart. So we see a type of "Ping-Pong effect" with each one activating the other. Imagine it this way, there is a room filled with mousetraps, loaded and lying on the floor. If we were to spring one mousetrap, that one trap would spring another, and that one would spring another, and the others would soon follow suit in a frenzied SNAP!

B cells and Antibodies: Gentle Soldiers

One way the immune system can differentiate harmful bacteria from harmless cells is by recognizing certain particles on their membranes or coatings. Like the particles that macrophages present on their cell membrane, antigens are also present on the intact pathogen. Certain cells of the immune system, called "B cells," contain receptors that are specific for these particles. These receptors are called "antibodies" and, when an antigen meets with its specific antibody on a B cell, the B cell becomes activated and begins to divide. After the B cell divides, antibody-secreting cells are created, which excrete more antibodies specific to the original antigen. Also created in the cloning are cells called memory cells that "remember" the pathogen and can survive for decades and produce specific antibodies for the rest of your life. Consequently, we only contract chicken pox once. After the initial attack, the body remembers the pathogen's "fingerprint" and can prevent further attacks.

Antibodies immobilize pathogens in several ways. They can simply surround the microorganism and effectively block it from doing harm. Antibodies can also bring several pathogens together into a group, making them more obtrusive and, therefore, easier for other immune cells to destroy. Perhaps the most significant role of the antibody is in activating a group of proteins called "complement." Complement can directly destroy microorganisms by forming into a tubular structure and inserting itself into the cell membrane of a pathogen, causing it to break apart. Complement can also coat microorganisms, making them easier to destroy by the phagocytes. The B cells and antibodies are the "gentle soldiers" of the body because they do not directly destroy microorganisms, but their overall effect is devastating to them. (See Figure 5.1.)

Natural Killer Cells

Yet another type of immune cell, the natural killer cell, is in charge of one specific task: destroying aberrant body cells. In the metaphor that introduced this chapter, a palace guard discovers a traitor in the castle. In our bodies natural killer cells seek out and destroy tumor cells and infected cells. It is important to state here that it is perfectly natural for the body to contain cancer cells and cells infected with many different types of viruses and bacteria. It is when these cells grow out of control that the trouble begins, and disease becomes imminent. Again, natural killer cells never eradicate aberrant cells completely, but they keep them in check. More specifically, natural killer cells do not engulf their prey, but rather cause the membrane of infected cells to tear, destroying the cell directly. Any lessening of their effectiveness, always possible during stress, can have serious implications for the health of the individual.

Supplementary Defenses

Other immune responses include the release of chemicals that raise the temperature in the body. A fever can make it difficult for many microorganisms to divide while increasing the phagocyte's ability to engulf cells and viruses. Clotting proteins help to heal wounds and seal off the area of infection, and blood itself can carry microorganisms away from the body. Another type of T cell, the suppressor T cell, calms the immune response down when the threat has passed.

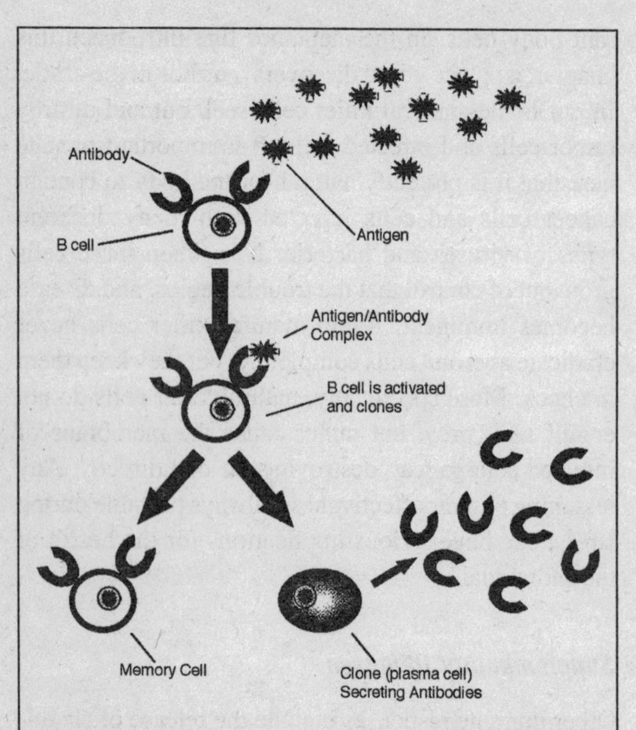

Figure 5.1 Cloning of B cells and creation of memory cells. The antibodies produced by the clone are specific to the original antigen. The memory cell may stay alive for decades, imparting to the individual lifetime resistance to the specific antigen.

Stress and the Immune System

It is an unfortunate fact that nearly 80 percent of all illness can be traced to stress. Furthermore, the American Academy of Family Physicians reports that almost two thirds of all medical office visits are prompted by stress. This being the case, it would seem a good idea to educate the public about the deleterious effects of stress, and to initiate far-reaching stress relief programs and workshops. Unfortunately, this is not being done, with medical schools themselves rarely touching on the subject. You can bet that every grade school student knows how to guard him- or herself against Lyme's disease, but stress—what grade school student has ever been instructed on how to deal with stress? In another light, while the mainstream medical community sometimes portrays meditation and other antistress techniques as unorthodox, their response to stress remains wanting. Clearly, the problem of stress, and the problems related to stress, are helping to destroy our society while costing us billions of unnecessary dollars in health care. Stress runs rampant in the modern day rat-race world, but it is also a silent killer, with little resistance mounted against it. Unlike bacteria, viruses, and even cancer, which our immune system can counteract and destroy in part, stress suppresses immunity and destroys our resistance to other forms of attack. This may be the key to how stress has been able to secure such a foothold in modern society; it kills by lowering resistance and allowing other opportunistic and degenerative diseases to flourish.

Stress affects the immune system for one very simple reason: energy conservation. When we are stressed, a great deal of the body's energy and resources are expended to restore balance in the body. For example, when humans are faced with the prospect of a charging tiger, the body goes into the so-called "fight or flight" mode, initiating a cascade of events that make great feats of speed and strength possible. But its benefits do not come without a cost. Put simply, energy is shuttled away from such systems as the immune system, so that more energy can go toward defending the life of the individual. In short spurts, the immune system is capable of handling the shift. The problem occurs when we are chronically exposed to stress that continually robs energy from other systems. The general effect is a lowered immune response and decreased health.

Another important aspect to remember is that the body doesn't make a distinction between the situations causing the stress; it sees only a rising need for energy. Therefore, a charging tiger, a flash quiz, or a flat tire is all the same to the stress centers of the body. What does count, on the other hand, is the individual's response to the stressor. One study conducted in 1991 and published in *Psychological Science* showed that certain detrimental effects of stress (such as increasing the number of suppressor-T cells) are seen only in people who are overly sensitive to stress. These "high reactor" types of people, who show adverse effects from stress such as higher heart rates, are in greater peril from stress than people better suited to handle stress. It's all in the way one reacts to stress; everyone has stress in his life, but the key to greater immune health is in learning how to deal without "overreacting," both mentally and physically. Adaptogens such as Rhodiola rosea can truly beef up any supplement protocol and provide well-needed defense for our immune systems.

The Immune Cell Assassin

Many scientific studies have been conducted showing the direct effect of stress on individual cells of the immune system. Certain chemicals released during the stress reaction, such as norepinephrine and epinephrine, have been shown to drastically suppress natural killer cells. The result?—lowering our defenses against cancer and viral infection. One theory even suggests that cancer begins in cells infected with viruses; the very cells that natural killer cells destroy. In another study where volunteers were exposed to a twelve-minute period of stress induced by the threat of electric shock, lower than normal values were found for their natural killer cells after the stress.

Researchers have also observed individuals with high-stress lifestyles, comparing them to well-matched control groups to chart immune response to certain vaccines. Since vaccines are typically inactive forms of viruses, a strong immune response to the vaccine will indicate a similarly healthy response to the real virus. In this study, researchers gave the influenza vaccine to subjects chosen from Alzheimer's disease caregivers (an extremely high-stress job). Immune response was then compared to subjects not engaged in such stressful activity. It was found that the caregivers had poorer antibody and T-cell response and a lower level of interleukin 1 than the control group.

It is well known that stress increases production of certain chemicals called glucocorticoids in the body. These chemicals function to raise the level of glucose in the blood, and, therefore, to increase available energy resources. Unfortunately, glucocorticoids also inhibit interleukin 2 and a chemical known as IFN–4. We have already discussed the function of interleukin 2 above; IFN–4 activates macrophages to engulf bacterial, viral, and tumor cells. Rising glucocorticoid levels have also been shown to lower the effectiveness of natural killer cells.

Stress and Resistance

Many studies have shown the deleterious effects that stress has on general immunity in the body. One study, for instance, found that medical students showed a higher risk of getting mononucleosis during examination periods than during less stressful times. Of course, other factors also could have infringed upon the immune system of these students at this time, such as sleep deprivation and poor nutrition. Investigators have also observed that women engaged in stressful activities demonstrated slower healing time, needing an average nine days longer to heal a small wound than control subjects. For their part, children exposed to high levels of stress were shown to have lowered immunity in their lungs than children who were not stressed. In sum, when we are stressed, we are much more likely to become infected with opportunistic viruses and bacteria, and our wound healing is delayed.

Rhodiola rosea—Diplomatic Immunity

The focus of this chapter thus far has been the immune system, and how stress affects it. Although the prognosis may seem rather bleak in the twentieth-century, high-stress world, help is in sight. For thousands of years, people all around the world have been using adaptogens (although the term "adaptogen" was not coined until 1947) to help their bodies deal with the effects of stress. Ancient cultures revered adaptogenic herbs for their balancing properties, but the need for such plants has probably never been so great as today.

Rhodiola rosea exerts a protective and stimulating

effect on the immune system in two major ways: by stimulating specific immune defenses, and by bringing the body closer to a state of homeostasis (biochemical balance). It has been shown above that many effects of stress diminish natural killer cell activity of the immune system. Rhodiola rosea may reverse this outcome. In one experiment, animals given Rhodiola rosea extract were shown to have increased natural killer cell activity in the gut and spleen. This increase may be due to Rhodiola rosea's ability to modulate glucocorticoid release into the body. Another study showed that extracts of Rhodiola rosea inhibited tumor growth in rats by 39 percent and decreased metastasis by 50 percent. Due to the natural killer cell's effect on tumors (more on cancer and Rhodiola rosea in Chapter 6). Rhodiola rosea may also support B cell immunity by preventing the suppression of B cell cloning which can occur during stress.

In its role as an adaptogen, Rhodiola rosea is the perfect antidote to the societal ills of increasing stress and decreased immunity. One of its most important roles in stress modulation is in bringing about homeostasis in the body. With homeostasis, immune cells function properly, and chemicals such as glucocorticoids and IFN–4 remain at levels consistent with health. When taken wisely, Rhodiola rosea normalizes the immune system and hormone levels in a positive way, bringing them into balance. In this way Rhodiola rosea can cut down on the harmful effects stress has on the immune system before they even occur. All adaptogenic herbs can help to relieve stress in the body and therefore exert some protective effect on the immune system, but Rhodiola rosea is the leader of the pack when it comes to specific immune enhancement. In short, Rhodiola rosea can be seen as a unique, balancing, antistress, immuno-protective herb well suited to become part of any modern herbal protocol.

Recommended Immune Support Formula

Standardized Rhodiola rosea	200 mg
Standardized Andrographis paniculata	200 mg
Standardized Astragalus	200 mg
Standardized Reishi Mushroom	100 mg
Standardized Shiitake Mushroom	100 mg
Standardized Cat's Claw	200 mg
Standardized Licorice	100 mg
Standardized Elderberry	200 mg
Standardized Echinacea	100 mg

Add a Comprehensive Antioxidant Formula to the herbal support above—take as directed on label.

CHAPTER 6

Rhodiola rosea and Cancer

The Basic Unit of Life

Cells are the most basic unit of life, the smallest functional structure capable of carrying out processes vital for survival. The entire body is a medley of different cells glued together and functioning synchronously like the proverbial "well-oiled machine." But cells eventually die. The cause of death—environmental toxins and excessive free-radicals that leave the cell irreparably damaged or viral infection that destroys the cell directly or signals the immune system to do the same. Or the cells just wear out because of age. Billions of cells are lost each day, but just as many are being born to take their predecessors places. Replacing old cells with new cells is possible because of a process called "mitosis," or cell division, and without it, we would slowly disappear, a billion cells at a time.

Mitosis: Two for the Price of One

Mitosis involves the separation of one "parent" cell into two identical "daughter" cells; "identical" being the key word here, both in form and function. A skin cell, for example, will always divide into two identical skin cells and not a liver cell or heart cell or brain cell. Perhaps the most important process in cell division is the replication of a very large and complex molecule called deoxyribonucleic acid or DNA (Figure 6.1). Deoxyribonucleic acid is the molecule of life, our hereditary history, coiled and compressed into a double helix in a space smaller than the head of a pin. It is what makes plants—plants, fish—fish, and people—people. Like a dictionary, DNA defines who you are, what you look like, how you talk and walk, and even how you behave. You are the product of your parents' DNA, mingling together and recombining in an almost infinite number of possibilities to produce you. You are what your DNA tells you what you are.

Division is a predictable and controlled process tightly regulated by environmental signals. Endocrine hormones, growth and differentiation factors, and stresses, such as heat, oxidation, and irradiation, initi-

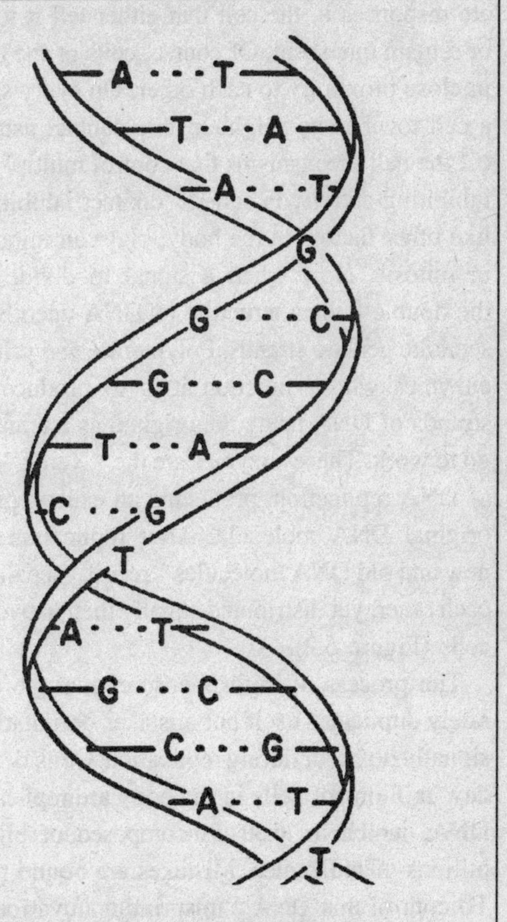

Figure 6.1 Double Helix Structure of the DNA Molecule

ate responses in the cell that either tell it to multiply or remain quiescent. Of course, cells of the body exist in close proximity to each other. On every side where a cell touches its neighbor, this contact usually turns off the cell mechanisms that control multiplying. This inhibiting activity is called "contact inhibition" and, like other factors in the body, plays an important role in mitosis. Now when a signal to divide is given, the double helical structure of DNA uncoils into two separate genetic strands. Polymerase and primase, two enzymes whose function it is to produce identical strands of DNA using the original as a template, then go to work. These enzymes are the "Xerox" machines of DNA replication, producing an exact replica of the original DNA molecule. After replication, both the new and old DNA molecules "recoil" separately from each other, yet distributed equally then in two daughter cells (Figure 6.2).

The process of mitosis ensures that the cell accurately duplicates itself but mistakes or mutations occasionally do occur during replication. Consider that each day, millions of cells in the body are replicating their DNA, which in itself, is composed of billions and billions of molecules. Mistakes are bound to happen. To control this DNA "misprinting," various mechanisms are available to the cell to correct the aberrant DNA or to destroy the cell altogether (a process called "programmed death") if the genetic flaw is irreparable. Despite their efforts though, DNA flaws do get past the checkpoints. A cell can then begin to multiply out of control and infiltrate the surrounding tissue. It is a process we well know. It is called cancer.

Cancer and the Cell: Programmed Madness

Cancer is a genetic disease that initiates in the cell and is characterized by: (1) cell growth not regulated by environmental factors, and (2) the cancerous cell's capacity to invade surrounding tissues. It is a disease of epidemic proportions, claiming more than 500,000 lives annually. Age has the most significant impact on cancer incidence and mortality, which doubles every five years after the age of twenty-five. Different types of cancer also reach different peaks during various times of the life cycle. For example, cancer of the colon, prostate, and stomach reach a peak incidence between 60 and 80 years. Of course, cancer is a systemic disease that has the capacity to develop in any tissue of the body.

As cancer cells divide, they accumulate, forming a mass known as a tumor. The tumor cells hoard nutrients and compete with healthy tissue for space, eventually killing off normal cells. Malignant cells do not conform to the law of contact inhibition; they grow out of control infiltrating the surrounding tissue even

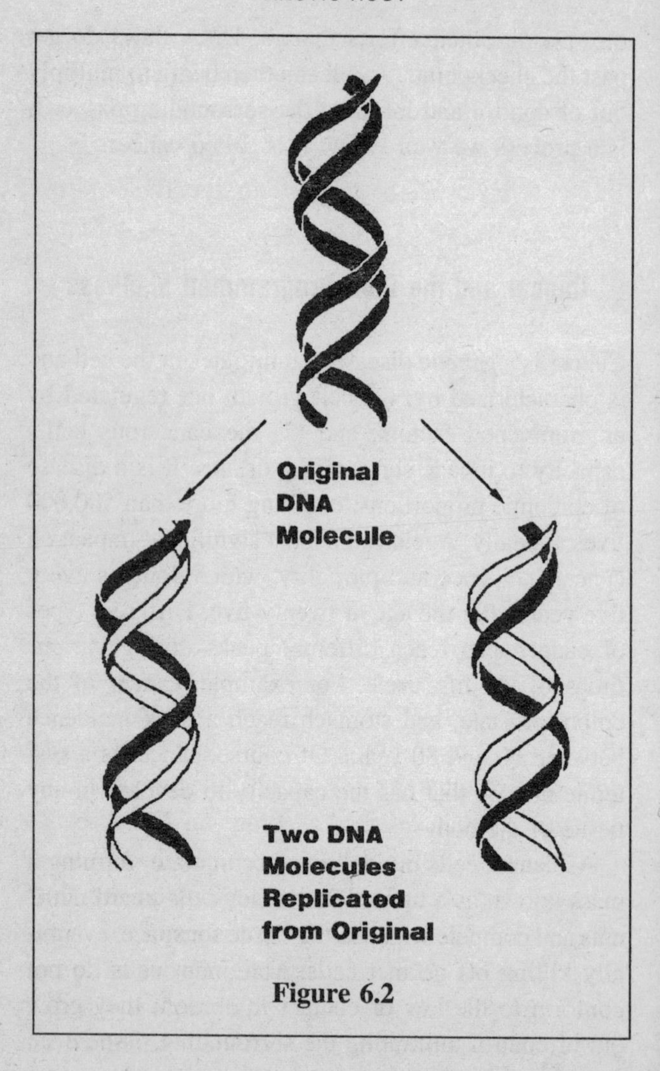
Original
DNA
Molecule
Two DNA
Molecules
Replicated
from Original

Figure 6.2

further. In the last phases of tumor development, the tumor becomes vascularized; that is, it produces its own network for blood supply, redirecting circulation away from healthy tissue. A healthy blood supply allow cells to break away from the tumor, travel through the blood and establish a new cancerous growth in another part of the body. This process is called "metastasis." Pain from cancer comes from tumor growth that applies pressure on nerves or blocks passageways, so that cellular and other secretions build up pressure.

Whatever the primary cause, cancer is not the result of a single insult but rather is a multistep process. As many as ten distinct mutations have to accumulate in a cell before it becomes cancerous, and these derangements may take up to several years before they become clinically evident. Although some forms of cancer are inheritable, most mutations are caused by carcinogenic exposure or by intrinsic errors in replication that affect specific regions on the DNA molecule called genes. Before, I said that the DNA molecule contains all the information that defines an organism. More specifically, DNA is composed of genes, the basic unit of heredity that occupies specific regions on the DNA molecule and defines the characteristics of the organism. There's a gene for every one of your attributes: blue eyes, black hair, big feet, you name it. There is also a class of genes that determine whether or not you develop cancer. They are called protooncogenes and oncogenes.

Protooncogenes are "normal" genes concerned with the regulation of cell proliferation. But these protooncogenes can mutate, leading to a gene that inappropriately perpetuates cell division. The protooncogenes is now called an oncogene, and it is the genetic basis underlying cancer. How protooncogenes mutate into cancerous oncogenes are a still a matter of speculation. Below are some purported mechanisms.

The Methods Behind Cancer's Madness

Every day we breath air, drink water, and eat food laden with pesticides and pollutants which contribute to DNA mutagenicity. Free radicals, which we have heard so much about lately, also play a part in DNA mutagenicity. In effect, free radicals are highly reactive molecules produced in the normal course of metabolism. Superoxide, hydrogen peroxide, and hydroxyl, a few of the many free radicals produced in the body, are also kept in check by the contrary forces of antioxidant enzymes—catalase, superoxide dismutase, and glutathione peroxidase, to name a few. Dietary antioxidants, including vitamins C and E and the provitamin betacarotene, also quench free radical activity. It is when free radical propagation outpaces antioxidant extinguishing that genetic damage may occur. DNA that is irreparably damaged by free radicals, for instance, usually initiates programmed cell death, thus stopping the possibility of replicating mutated DNA molecules. But free radical damage that does not initiate programmed cell death can stimulate the development of cancer. Additionally, catecholamines may undergo "autoxidation" that produces free radicals. But whether antioxidation contributes to the formation of cancer still remains to be seen.

Viral infections have also fallen under the objective eye of science as a possible cause of cancer. Viruses are tiny packages of genetic material that can insert their genes into our DNA, turning our cells into mirror-like virus-producing factories. How viruses actually contribute to cancer is still speculative, but science has postulated that viruses may insert their own protooncogenes or oncogenes into the host's DNA, thereby increasing the likelihood of a cell turning to a life of uncontrollable division. Although the clinical evidence of viruses causing many types of cancer is scant, there are a few types of cancer that may have their roots in viral infection (Table 6.1).

Just as there are genes to stimulate cell division, there are also genes to suppress replication, the "tumor-suppressing genes." These genes work by either halting the replication process or initiating cell suicide if the DNA is damaged. The P53 gene, also known as "the guardian of the genome," is a gene well

Table 6.1 Viruses That May Cause Cancer

Viruses That May Cause Cancer
Papillomavirus
Cytomegalovirus
Epstein-Barr virus
Hepatitis B
Human T–Lymphotropic virus–1

known to suppress cellular division. Genetic damage or mutations, however, may lead to alteration in P53, suppressing the suppressor and allowing a cell with aberrant DNA to divide out of control.

Investigations into psychoneuroimmunology, or the study of the relationship between emotions and the immune response, suggest that stress, although it does not directly cause cancer, may contribute to it by activating latent cancer cells or by suppressing the immune system as a whole.

Stress and the Cancer Connection

The immune system, of course, is cancer's most formidable enemy. The process by which the immune system surveys for and destroys cancerous cells is analogous to the process of the body rejecting transplanted tissues. The body "sees" cancerous cells as non-self and mobilizes lymphocytes, macrophages, and natural killer cells to destroy the offending party. As we have seen in the previous chapter, stress may suppress the activity of natural killer cells and other cells involved in cancer cell destruction. With a suppressed immune system, cancer cells have an open invitation to proliferate and infiltrate.

Chronic stress in humans can also change the biochemical mechanisms in a cell, turning it to anaerobic metabolism instead of aerobic metabolism. For a cell to produce energy efficiently, oxygen must be present; this process is known as aerobic respiration. In its absence, the cell can still produce energy although somewhat less efficiently. In this condition the cell is said to be operating under anaerobic (without oxygen) conditions. Under normal circumstances a sufficient amount of oxygen is present to carry out aerobic respiration and carry out efficient energy production. What is the connection to stress? When exposed to a stressful situation, the cell may switch from aerobic respiration to anaerobic, even in the presence of adequate oxygen! At this point, the unused oxygen becomes toxic to the cell and causes DNA damage. To compensate, cellular enzymes attempt to repair the damaged DNA by replicating new DNA. The continual attempts of the enzymes to replace sections of damaged DNA leads to such mutations that the cell eventually becomes cancerous and even worse, metastatic.

Undoubtedly, there are several mechanisms involved in cancer and to effectively fight it we need to address cancer on multiple levels. Unfortunately, many of the drugs used to combat cancer are singular in their purpose. Some are effective only during cell division and may be ineffective against the majority of tumor cells that are not multiplying. Chemotherapy does not address prevention for example, but is employed only after the cancer has established itself. Ironically, the drugs used in chemotherapy may be just as lethal as the cancer itself, a sort of ''kill before being killed'' mentality that can result in severe abnormalities, including liver dysfunction, inflammation and ulceration of the mucous membranes, anemia, suppressed immune system, and the list goes on. As far as Western medicine is concerned, chemotherapy and radiation are the state-of-the-art treatments for treating cancer. But unbeknownst to them, a plant growing wild in the polar arctic regions of Russia may prove to be a viable alternative or adjunct to conventional therapies.

Rhodiola rosea: Combating Cancer Naturally

Decades before the West was privy to the beneficial effects of Rhodiola rosea, Soviet scientists, behind the veil of the iron curtain, studied this herb's potent anticarcinogenic properties. Here is what they found:

- Oral administration of Rhodiola rosea improved the characteristics of urothelial tissue and immunity in patients suffering from superficial bladder cancer. Investigators also found that the average frequency of relapse in the Rhodiola rosea group fell twice, although it was not statistically significant.
- In animals suffering from Pliss lymphosarcoma, it was shown that extracts of Rhodiola rosea inhibited the growth of tumors by 50 percent and when combined with a partial hepatectomy, inhibition rose to 75 percent. In the combined treatment group, the process of liver regeneration was completed in an earlier time span as compared to animals that had undergone partial hepatectomy only.
- In another experiment, mice suffering from various types of cancer, including adenocarcinoma (malignant cancer of glandular tissue) and lung carcinoma were given extracts of Rhodiola rosea that resulted in an increased survival rate.

Rhodiola rosea, living up to the criterion of being nonspecific, affects cancer, both before and after it has established and gained a foothold. The antioxidant properties of Rhodiola rosea have been extensively studied and shown to be enormously high as compared to other natural antioxidants. Lipid peroxidation, for example, is the process by which lipids go rancid and occurs when oxygen and free radicals react with fatty acids, destroying their chemical structure. Lipid peroxidation, therefore, is a good indicator of free radical and antioxidant activity. Researchers examined the activity of lipid peroxidation processes in the small intestines under acute irradiation (a potent generator of free radicals). When exposed to radiation, structural alterations and elevated lipid peroxidation levels were seen. A preparation containing a dry extract of Rhodiola rosea produced a strong antiperoxidation effect on lipid membranes; that is, it protected lipid membranes from free radical attack. It can be concluded that Rhodiola rosea may protect against cancer by sparing sensitive cell structures from the sting of free radicals.

To confirm Rhodiola rosea's effectiveness in preventing mutations, alcoholic extracts of the herb were employed in the Ames test, a procedure that evaluates the carcinogenicity of chemicals. Using 20 percent and 40 percent alcoholic extracts, Rhodiola rosea was tested for its ability to suppress the capacity of mutagenic compounds that may induce malignant changes in DNA. Rhodiola rosea was shown to suppress genetic mutations; this effect was particularly pronounced in the 40 percent extract solution. **Rhodiola rosea com-**

pletely suppressed the activity of weak mutagens and attenuated the activity of moderate mutagens by 80 to 92 percent.

Rhodiola rosea may actively participate in not only preventing free radical and mutagen damage, but it may also repair damage that has already been done. Researchers, studying the effects of N–nitroso–N–Methylurea (NMU) and cyclophosphamide (ironically used in cancer therapy) on DNA aberrations in bone marrow cells, found that Rhodiola rosea significantly reduced the number of DNA alterations caused by these two compounds. They concluded that extracts of Rhodiola rosea are antimutagens due to their ability to raise the efficiency of DNA repair mechanisms. Finally, Rhodiola rosea may slow the progression of cancer when concentrations of the herb demonstrated marked ability to prevent the growth and proliferation of cells. It is clear that Rhodiola rosea's potential to combat cancer is promising and, when used in combination with conventional therapies, may provide a greater therapeutic outcome without the associated side effects from chemotherapy.

The antibiotic adriamycin is a popular drug used in cancer therapy but may result in pronounced liver dysfunction. When used in combination with Rhodiola rosea, the toxic effects of the drug are attenuated. In fact, when used in combination, both Rhodiola rosea and adriamycin proved to be very powerful against metastasis.

Pharmacological treatments are a cutting-edge technology in the United States, but their search for a "magic bullet" has been in vain. The "one disease—one cure" paradigm of modern medicine has blinded us to a host of natural products that may be just as effective. The medical community has been lulled into believing that in order to treat disease, drugs must be used. Pharmaceutical industries, not seeing any financial gain, commonly ignore the possibilities that natural products have to offer. In a manner of speaking, Rhodiola rosea may be the magic bullet we are looking for. Instead of a single magic bullet, I prefer the analogy of a shotgun with many tiny bullets spreading out in all directions.

Recommended Anti-Cancer Support Formula

Standardized Rhodiola rosea	200 mg
Beta 1,3 Glucans	200 mg
D–Limonene	100 mg
Modified Citrus Pectin	1 g
Soy Isoflavones	100 mg
Indole-3–Carbinol	200 mg
Quercetin	300 mg
Lutein	15 mg
Lycopene	15 mg
Calcium D–Glucarate	1 g

To be taken with a comprehensive Antioxidant Formula and Immune Support Formula—as directed on the label.

CHAPTER 7

Rhodiola rosea and Human Performance

The Performance Connection

Russia's world class athletes well know how their successes are tied up with use of Rhodiola rosea. In fact, the majority of scientific research on Rhodiola rosea is geared toward enhancing physical and mental performance whether it is of an extreme or ordinary nature. Human performance, of course, is an eclectic term that can mean different things for different people in different situations. Simply walking or climbing stairs could be considered as intense a physical exertion for an elderly individual, as an Olympic wrestling event is for a trained professional. Mental exertion during the workday could also be as equally taxing to the person behind the desk as it would be for the professional chess player competing against peers. In this chapter we explore Rhodiola rosea's ability to enhance physical and mental performance for the professional athlete who trains eight hours a day and for the rest of us who try to survive eight hours a day.

Exercise and Stress: Another Side of the Same Coin

Exercise is a stress, but along with diet and lifestyle, it does have its place in health. Exercise enhances the body's ability to burn fat while increasing lean body mass. Emotional and physical strength and posture improve with regular physical activity. Cardiovascular functioning becomes more efficient, allowing the heart to work less and accomplish more. Finally, regular exercise plays an integral part in preventing disease, such as osteoporosis, heart disease, hypertension, cancer, and diabetes. The similarities between both physical and psychological stress lie in their ability to induce the same response. Physical exertion initiates a cascade of compensatory reactions to resist the forces applied to the body. It stimulates the immediate mobilization of energy mediated through the sympathetic nervous system and adrenal glands, thus intensifying energy expenditure and oxygen consumption in skeletal and heart muscle.

But unlike the burden of psychological stress, exercise initiates its own adaptive processes. Physical stress, like that experienced when exercising or when fighting off an attacker, is quite different from the passive and beguiling psychological stress that we are exposed to every day. The salient difference here is that physical stress initiates its own adaptive processes, making the organism better suited to deal with similar, future stresses. Environmental and psychological stress, on the other hand, burdens us in many ways. Quite simply, **the body cannot adapt to psychological and environmental stress.** Compound this problem with the fact that exercise is more of a concept than a lifestyle, something we think about more than we do, and we can see why illness is running rampant in our society.

So, in a matter of speaking, the body doesn't become stronger because of exercise, it becomes better adapted. It's what professional athletes strive for and, in their efforts, have turned to various substances—some legal, others illegal—to get the edge they need to stay on top. The many studies investigating Rhodiola rosea's effects during athletic performance may provide the answer that athletes have sought:

- Based on data obtained from observations on weightlifters, wrestlers, and gymnasts, extracts of Rhodiola rosea increased physical work capacity, decreased fatigue, and improved the general mental and physical state of the subjects.

- Using 112 athletes, researchers discovered that 89 percent of those supplementing with Rhodiola rosea showed a more rapid improvement in performance in sports such as track and field, swimming, speed skating, and ski racing. Speed and strength qualities of the tested individuals improved in comparison to the control group. Researchers also revealed that out of those supplementing Rhodiola rosea, 69 percent displayed accelerated adaptation to climatic and social conditions, and 86 percent demonstrated improved appetite. This study further solidified Rhodiola's influence on the rehabilitative processes in professional athletes.
- The influence of a preparation of adaptogens, including Rhodiola, on work capacity and functional state of the cardiovascular system of healthy individuals during intense and prolonged physical loads in low temperatures were investigated. The study employed highly qualified skiers during training races and during a biathlon that required the athletes to ski for 12 miles while carrying a rifle and shooting at halts. The subjects who received the adaptogen preparation had better technical results for distance and a significantly greater number of strikes on target shooting at halts. Thirty minutes after completing the competition, the heart rates in both the Rhodiola rosea and control group were recorded. Heart rate can be used to assess the level of recovery after a

physical load and thus serve as an indicator of adaptation. In the Rhodiola rosea group, heart rate was 104 to 106 percent that of baseline. In the control group, heart rate was 128.7 percent. The adaptogenic preparation containing Rhodiola rosea proved effective in enhancing physical performance and hastening the recovery process.

- In 52 individuals, ages 18 to 24 years, a preparation including Rhodiola rosea proved to enhance the duration of physical performance by 12 percent. Amazingly, work performance increased to 28 percent after the test subjects were initially fatigued and then asked to perform the test.
- When compared to anabolic steroids, researchers discovered that Rhodiola rosea had a comparable effect without the negative effects on the function of the adrenal glands.

The Mechanics of Rhodiola rosea

Based on these studies and the multitude that have been performed in the former Soviet Union, scientists and trainers have recommended Rhodiola rosea in many areas of athletic performance for improving speed and strength abilities and for enhancing the recovery process. But even in their bolstering, researchers are still unsure how Rhodiola rosea

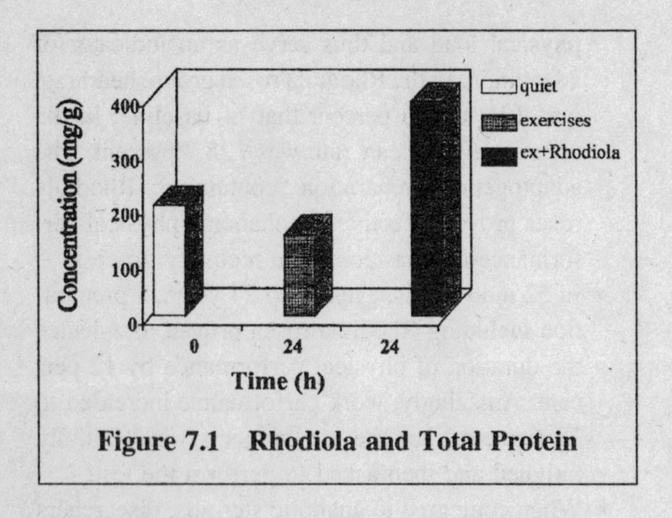

Figure 7.1 Rhodiola and Total Protein

enhances physical performance. But then again, how does a scientist specifically explain something that works nonspecifically?

Throughout the years, many have pondered Rhodiola rosea's ability to enhance physical performance. Many have demonstrated Rhodiola rosea's anabolic effects, including the capacity to increase body weight by improving the muscle-fat ratio and increasing hemoglobin and erythrocyte levels. Muscle proteins and glutamic acid are also enhanced when supplementing with Rhodiola rosea (Figures 7.1 and 7.2).

Glutamic acid is a derivative of glutamine, an amino acid found in muscle and participates in muscle metabolism by removing nitrogenous waste and acting as a

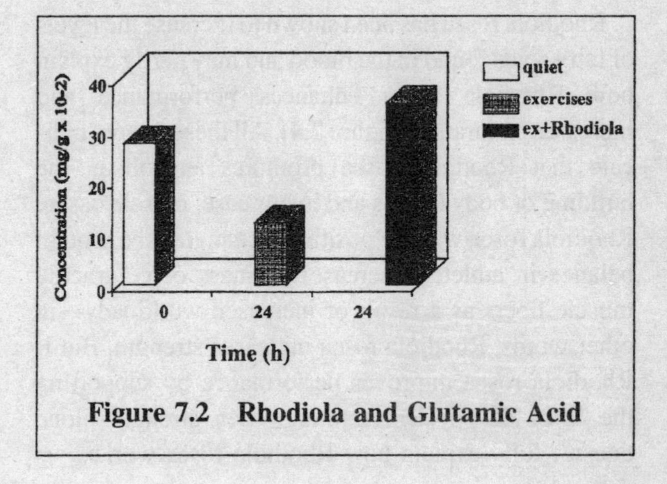

Figure 7.2 Rhodiola and Glutamic Acid

substrate for glucose synthesis as well as the synthesis of other amino acids. Glutamic acid may preserve muscle mass since low levels of this amino acid are associated with decreased muscle mass.

Other compounds critical for muscular performance are creatine phosphate and adenosine triphosphate (ATP), both of which are the muscle's primary energy molecules. Rhodiola rosea has been shown to increase muscle ATP and creatine phosphate levels (Figure 7.3). In addition to using glucose for ATP production, the body mobilizes fatty acid stores during prolonged exercise. In fact, fatty acids play a greater role in supporting the energy demands of the body during long-term exercise than glucose alone.

Rhodiola rosea has been shown to increase the levels of fatty acids found in the blood and may partly explain how Rhodiola rosea enhances performance and increases endurance (Figure 7.4). All these factors indicate that Rhodiola rosea promotes anabolism, the building of body tissues and in our case, muscle tissue. Rhodiola rosea will, by positively changing the protein balance in athletes, increase the mass of contractile muscle fibers as a result of increased workloads—in other words, Rhodiola rosea increases strength. But if Rhodiola rosea improves performance by supporting the level of physical training, then strength alone doesn't fully explain how Rhodiola rosea works.

Rhodiola rosea and the Dichotomy of Performance

Physical performance is dichotomous and understanding how Rhodiola rosea enhances strength only partially explains how it enhances performance. Rhodiola rosea plays a much broader role, a role that keeps it in line with its primary effect in the body—adaptogenic. Remember; Exercise is a stress and, thus, requires adaptation by the body; the adaptation process requires a system to regulate it and reserves to fuel it.

It's no surprise that the same systems that regulate the stress response also regulate our response to exercise. The sympathetic nervous system (SNS) is the most important regulator needed to mobilize energy

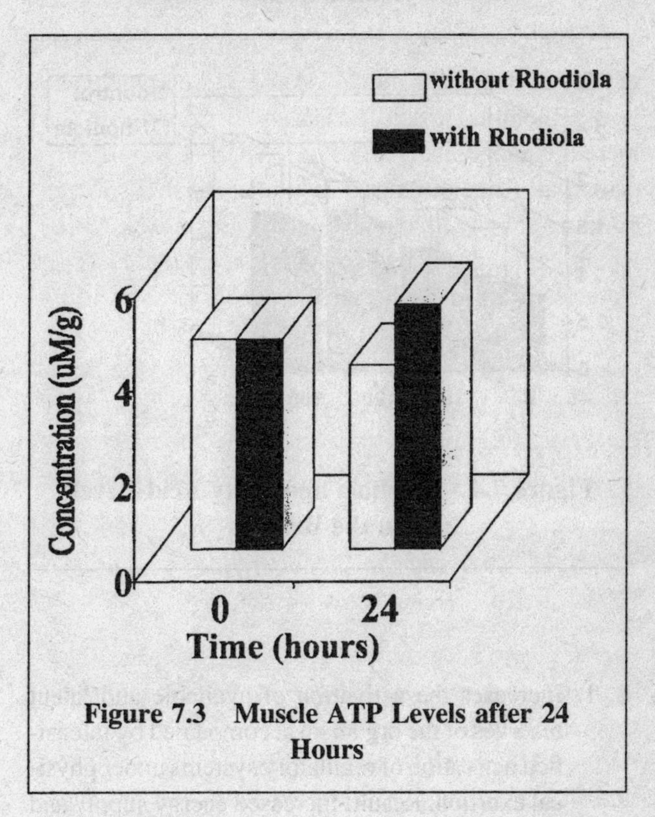

Figure 7.3 Muscle ATP Levels after 24 Hours

and metabolic reserves against fatigue. It accomplishes this by one of three ways:

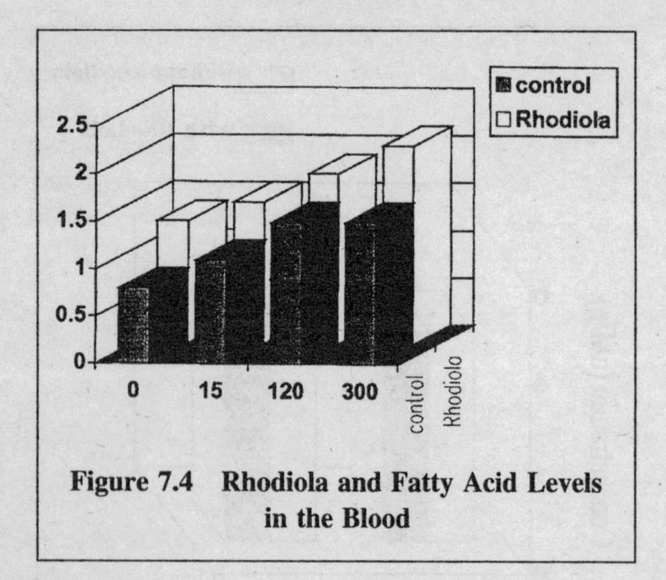

Figure 7.4 Rhodiola and Fatty Acid Levels in the Blood

1. Increases the activation of available and latent reserves of the organism accompanied by intensified activation of regulatory systems under physical exertion. Result: Increased energy supply and sympathetic nervous stimulation.
2. Makes more economical use of functional reserves when exertion of the regulatory system during the physical load should decrease or remain unchanged. Result: More efficient use of metabolic reserves in the face of decreased autonomic stimulation.

3. Increases functional reserves as a result of regular physical training when exertion of the regulatory systems should be reduced. Result: Training induces a more economical use of reserves than in nontrained individuals in whom even low physical exertion induces considerable exertion of the regulatory system.

So, in order to increase endurance we must increase the mobilization of metabolic reserves as well as the activity of the sympathetic nervous system, provide more efficient use of reserves during decreased SNS stimulation, or increase metabolic reserves which normally occurs during regular physical activity. In order to increase physical performance, we must increase the activity of the SNS or mobilization of metabolic reserves or both. With a deficiency in one, there is an overstimulation of the other.

When metabolic reserves are low, the regulatory system must work harder to adapt to the physical stress. Conversely, the exertion of the regulatory system decreases if reserves are high. Therefore, the level of physical performance is determined by the capacity of the metabolic reserve. Rhodiola rosea enhances performance by decreasing the level of exertion of the regulatory system under physical stress, thus reducing the "price of adaptation."

One way Rhodiola rosea does this is by activating the parasympathetic nervous system (PNS). The SNS and PNS are diametrically opposed, the former stimulating and the latter relaxing. Researchers have shown that subjects supplementing with Rhodiola rosea initially had a rise in SNS activity, but as the experiment continued, a gradual increase in PNS activity became apparent. Prolonged overstimulation of the SNS may signify the body's inability to adapt, and the inability to adapt results in fatigue. Activation of the parasympathetic nervous system demonstrates Rhodiola rosea's ability to induce adaptation, sparing the body from prolonged SNS stimulation and the fatigue that follows. Researchers also speculate that Rhodiola rosea decreases the level of regulatory system exertion by promoting a more efficient use of metabolic reserves and/or mobilizing additional reserves without intensifying SNS activity.

Rhodiola rosea seems to be a powerful supplement that could enhance performance in today's top athletes. But what about the nine-to-five masses—those of us who run for the bus instead of running for health? It seems that Rhodiola rosea is equally as effective in the corporate executive and construction foreman as it is in highly trained athletes.

Extracts of Rhodiola rosea have proven to be a valuable therapeutic agent in apparently healthy individuals with a tendency toward asthenia during work. Asthenia is a psychosomatic disorder characterized by mental and physical fatigue, dyspnea (labored breathing), giddiness, precordial pain (pain in the chest), and palpitations. It occurs in individuals exposed to stressful conditions, especially intense mental demands. Asthenia at work results in higher absenteeism rates and decreased worker performance. To test Rhodiola rosea's anti-asthenic properties, 27 healthy students, physicians, and scientific workers, ages 19 to 46 years, were prescribed extracts derived from the plant. The protocol consisted of 100 milligrams, taken morning and afternoon for two to three weeks. Extracts of Rhodiola rosea were also administered several days before anticipated intensified intellectual work and throughout the period of intellectual strain. In all cases, the Rhodiola rosea extract prevented asthenic decompensation during intense mental performance.

In another study, a desired therapeutic effect was obtained with patients exhibiting symptoms of asthenic syndrome. Symptoms of muscle weakness, constant sluggishness, hypersomnia (excessive sleeping), low motivational levels, and apathy declined after the administration of 100 to 150 milligrams of Rhodiola rosea extract. Their symptoms decreased so much that the researchers were able to decrease their dosages to 50 milligrams per day. In an experiment conducted on 52 workers carrying out intense physical labor, a preparation containing Rhodiola rosea administered prior to their workload demonstrated marked improvement in their general and mental state. Functional indicators including pulse, arterial pressure, back muscle strength, hand strength endurance, and coordination of movement improved. After the workload, workers experienced quicker recovery time.

Rhodiola rosea and Memory

Several studies have demonstrated Rhodiola rosea's ability to enhance a person's ability for memorization and prolonged concentration. In a proofreading test, those taking Rhodiola rosea extract decreased the number of their mistakes by 88 percent, while those in the control group, *increased* the number of their mistakes by 84 percent!

Another study was conducted using a proofreading test based on the so-called "Anfimov table." The Anfimov table offers the possibility of obtaining comparative results that characterize the quality and quantity of work performed. One-hundred-twenty students, 20 to 28 years, performed the test twice, once before and again one hour after taking the Rhodiola rosea preparation. The control group received a solution similar in appearance to the solution given to the treatment group but lacking extracts of Rhodiola rosea. The difference in the number of symbols corrected in five minutes, before and after taking Rhodiola rosea, served as a quantitative measure of the herb. A change in the percent errors made in the process characterized the quality of work performed.

The results clearly demonstrate Rhodiola rosea's ability to enhance intellectual function. In the control groups, the change in the number of symbols corrected after one hour was insignificant, while the percent of errors made increased. In the treatment group, Rhodiola rosea exerted a stimulating effect on intellectual activity. In 84 to 88 percent of the subjects taking Rhodiola rosea, the number of symbols corrected increased by five to seven percent, while the number of errors made decreased by three to five percent. The quality of work performed was dependent on fatigue that set in during the study and Rhodiola rosea effectively increased a person's resistance to fatigue.

To test the duration of Rhodiola rosea's effect, investigators observed the treatment group one, two, three, four, six, eight and twenty-four hours after taking ten drops of the preparation. When compared to the control group Rhodiola rosea's effects are astonishing. After one hour, those taking a placebo experienced a 13 percent increase in the number of errors made. By the fourth hour, the number of errors increased by 37 percent; at the sixth hour there was an 88 percent increase; and by the eighth hour, a whopping 180 percent increase was observed. In the Rhodiola rosea group, a 56 percent decrease in the number of errors was observed, and this effect lasted four hours. After that, the percent of errors made increased but to a lesser extent than in the control group. The investigators concluded the preparation of Rhodiola rosea improves intellectual work capacity after a one-time dose; this effect is seen primarily in the quality of work performed.

Exactly how Rhodiola rosea influences learning and memory is still a topic of debate. According to contemporary notions, the process of memory formation is supported by the interactions between various chemical transmitters in the brain. The role of cholinergic (acetylcholine-activated neurons) transmission during the learning process and the formation of memory is well known but other transmitters in the brain are also important. The roles of different transmitter systems may be different depending on the nature of the learning process. As an example, in some animal experiments in which serotonin levels have been reduced, no significant changes in the learning process were shown, while other animal experiments have shown improved status. A few researchers have found that a moderate decrease of norepinephrine (noradrenaline) improves the learning and memory processes. Subsequent studies have shown that salidroside, one active found in Rhodiola rosea extracts, moderately lowers the amount of norepinephrine and dopamine in the brain. Because norepinephrine plays a critical role in the stress response and Rhodiola rosea can effectively modulate levels of this catecholamine, the latter theory may explain how this herb influences intellectual capacity. Additional studies are needed to fully elucidate the phenomenon between Rhodiola and memory.

Recommended Daily Pre- & Post-Exercise Formula

Standardized Rhodiola rosea	200 mg
Standardized American Ginseng	100 mg
Standardized Korean Ginseng	100 mg
Standardized Siberian Ginseng	100 mg
Coenzyme Q–10	100 mg
Lipoic Acid	100 mg
Creatine Monohydrate	2.5 g

Comprehensive Antioxidant Formula—as per label directions

Comprehensive B Complex—as per label directions

CHAPTER 8

Rhodiola rosea and Miscellaneous Marvels

Rhodiola rosea—A Bargain

We are creatures of habit. We are also creatures of bargains. Everything from the blue light special to "you get all this for only four easy payments of $99.99," we clamor to get as much as we can for as little as possible. We would gladly turn over our children for a television that cooks, cleans, and cuts the lawn, but there's an old saying, "you get what you pay for," and so not all bargains are as good as they may seem . . . except for one. Rhodiola rosea is nature's "blue light special," that continues to amaze science with its growing list of benefits. Oh and by the way, you can get it for a lot less than $99.99.

Sex and Rhodiola rosea: Now that I Have Your Attention . . .

For centuries, the roots of Rhodiola rosea were used as a powerful stimulant and favored ingredient in many folk love potions. The legendary Ukrainian prince Danila Galitsky (thirteenth century), who had remarkable amorous feats, boasted of strength coming from Rhodiola rosea. In the former Soviet Union, a favorite form of the herb is a tincture called ''nastojka,'' prepared by combining the fresh roots of Rhodiola rosea with 40 percent alcohol and allowing the mixture to sit for one week. A teaspoon of the resulting ''nastojka'' after breakfast, lunch, and dinner is prescribed for both men and women experiencing sexual disturbances.

Anecdotal reports of Rhodiola rosea's effectiveness against sexual dysfunction was put to the test when Russian scientists used the adaptogen in 35 men suffering from weak erections, premature ejaculation, or a combination of the two for one to twenty years. In addition to their primary condition, the patients also complained of increased irritability, excitability, poor sleep, and sweatiness. For three months, the subjects supplemented their regular diet with 50 milligrams of Rhodiola rosea. At the end of the treatment cycle a substantial improvement was seen in 26 out of 35 patients—that's 74 percent! Both the normalization of prostate fluid and an increase in 17–ketosteroids in the urine were noted by researchers. Seventeen–ketosteroids are used as an indicator of male hormone production in the body. Further experiments demonstrated that Rhodiola rosea is not gender biased. The effect of Rhodiola rosea on the functioning of sex glands served as another experiment in women suffering from amenorrhea.

The absence of the menstrual cycle is characteristic of amenorrhea and can be either one of two types: primary or secondary. The absence of menarche by age 16 is classified as primary amenorrhea, while the absence of menstruation for more than three months in women past menses is considered secondary amenorrhea. Forty women were chosen to participate in a study using Rhodiola rosea. For five months to five years or greater, these women suffered from either primary (7) or secondary amenorrhea (33). Some study group members were prescribed a 100 to 150 mg dose of Rhodiola rosea extract, twice a day for two weeks; others were given a one-milliliter injection of rhodosine for 10 days. After the course of treatment, investigators found that in 25 of the women suffering from secondary amenorrhea, the menstrual cycle resumed. Out of the 25 women whose menstrual cycle was restored, 11 became pregnant. This Valentine's Day, instead of chocolates and flowers, celebrate your relationship over a glass of nastojka.

Rhodiola rosea and Hearing: Listening to What Science Has to Say

The influence of extracts of Rhodiola rosea on the function of the hearing organ was also studied. Nineteen healthy individuals working in an electromechanical production plant and three pilots at a Soviet airport were included in the study. Before the administration of Rhodiola, a decrease in bone and air conduction for speech tones was identified in all subjects. Air and bone conduction are measurements of hearing made through either earphones (air) or through a vibrator placed on the mastoid bone behind the ear (bone). A lower conduction reading correlates to a decrease in auditory function (i.e., hearing). Subjects received 100 milligrams of Rhodiola rosea extract twice daily for two weeks. During the test period, air and bone conduction for speech tones had increased by ten to forty decibels in all 22 subjects two weeks after taking Rhodiola rosea extract daily. How Rhodiola rosea increases auditory function is still speculative but may be mediated through the herb's ability to enhance serotonin levels in the brain. Studies have shown that serotonin administered directly into the brain exerts a substantial influence on processes that increase the brain's reactivity to sensory stimulation.

Rhodiola rosea and Dentistry: Taking a Bite Out of Gum Disease

Rhodiola rosea extract has been used in dental practice for swabbing the gums of patients with pyorrhea, a gum disease characterized by the progression of gingivitis to the point that loss of supporting bone has begun. Pyorrhea is the primary cause of tooth loss in adults. A positive effect has been achieved from applications of Rhodiola rosea extract dissolved in water, in combination with retinol acetate (vitamin A). After four to seven days of treatment, gum hemorrhaging decreased, swelling diminished, and normal coloring was seen. Maybe we should be brushing our teeth with Rhodiola rosea instead of those chemical cocktails called toothpaste!

Rhodiola rosea and Blood Sugar: A Sweet Deal

Normally, the control of blood sugar is the responsibility of the pancreas. When we consume a meal rich in carbohydrates (or candies or sugary drinks), blood sugar levels rise, signaling special cells in the pancreas, called beta-cells, to produce and secrete insulin. Insulin is the most important hormone involved in regulating blood sugar. It is the body's ''doorman,'' clearing the blood of excess sugar by ushering it into the cells for energy production or storage as glycogen. In normal individuals a rise in glucose after a meal is normal, so long as it is followed by a gradual decline back to normal fasting levels. A persistent elevation in blood sugar is termed diabetes, the most common endocrine disorder in people.

Diabetes is a disorder of sugar metabolism because of a lack of insulin production or a loss in insulin's effectiveness. Without insulin, glucose cannot enter into cells and accumulates in the blood. As a result, blood sugar skyrockets. The body, in a desperate attempt to control the high levels, shuttles glucose off into alternative metabolic pathways or dumps excess sugar into the kidneys for excretion. The cells, deprived of their primary energy molecule, signal to the brain that they are starving and so the brain initiates the hunger response. As a result of these processes, the person urinates excessively and constantly drinks fluids to satiate thirst. They are constantly eating despite the fact they are losing weight. If left untreated, diabetes leads to complications of the cardiovascular system, kidneys, nervous system, and eyes. Alone, diabetes is an insidious disease, but when combined with stress, the two are a ticking bomb waiting to go off.

While there is little evidence supporting stress-induced diabetes, there is strong evidence that psychological stress can worsen the symptoms in preexisting diabetes. The effects of stress can once again be attributable to the stress response and the outpouring of hormones that work against insulin. Remember, the body cannot distinguish between different stresses; it just sees them all as one big threat and, so, mobilizes energy reserves to support action. Therefore, instead of storing glucose for future use, the body secretes stress hormones which result in a surge of glucose into a circulatory system that is already burdened with excess sugar. In addition to psychological stress exacerbating the complications associated with diabetes, stress reputedly leads to a progression of the disease by stimulating the destruction of beta cells. But there is a substance that may alleviate diabetes and the subsequent complications associated with it.

Rhodiola rosea not only decreases the levels of stress hormones in the body, a phenomenon we have seen time and time again, but it may also influence beta-cell activity. In animal experiments, researchers demonstrated Rhodiola rosea's hypoglycemic effects. Upon closer evaluation, they found that Rhodiola rosea raised blood insulin levels and decreased the levels of glucagon (an insulin antagonist). The administration of Rhodiola rosea also led to a 50 percent to 80 percent increase in liver glycogen, the main storage organ for blood sugar.

Rhodiola rosea and Aging

Perhaps the fountain of youth wasn't a fountain at all but a plant that grows in Siberia. Science has vigorously pursued the aging process in an attempt to slow it down but it's a race against the clock. Even though the chase has somewhat explained why cells age we are still powerless to stop it. Among the torrent of theories on aging, one that is noteworthy is the cortisol connection. Researchers have observed that aging in several marine species and an animal model is triggered by a large increase in cortisol due to stress. Cortisol is a glucocorticoid that is crucial in the response to trauma, infection, exercise, anxiety, and dementia. But high levels may cause involution of the thymus, depression of the immune response, tissue damage, fat deposition, confusion, and dementia. Within the blood, cortisol is normally bound to a protein called "cortisol-binding globulin and albumin." Although cortisol-binding globulin has a higher infinity for cortisol than albumin, overall, albumin transports a majority of the hormone in the blood. Thus, low levels of albumin, such as seen in premature infants and elderly individuals, may cause a rise in free cortisol and accelerated aging. Rhodiola rosea's adrenal-modulating activity may explain its antiaging effects but more research in this area is needed.

Rhodiola rosea and the Liver: Protecting the Protector

Among its many functions, the liver is an important organ involved in metabolizing toxins and medications to less damaging substances. But in its efforts to protect the body from harm, the liver itself may become a victim of toxic exposure. Rhodiola rosea may afford protection to the liver as demonstrated in its ability to prevent carbon tetrachloride intoxication. Carbon tetrachloride is a potent poison to the liver that could lead to chemically induced hepatitis. As we have seen in the chapter on cancer (Chapter 6), Rhodiola rosea may ameliorate the side effects associated with chemotherapy as well.

Toxicity and Dosage

It is worth noting that Rhodiola rosea is safer than Korean ginseng even in high doses. Although the majority of studies revealed no toxic side effects, some have reported increased arterial pressure, squeezing pains in the region of the heart behind the sternum with radiation to the left arm and scapula. The pains appeared more often in persons with a tendency toward coronary spasm and fluctuations in arterial pressure. Rhodiola rosea extract is contraindicated if the individual is experiencing nervous excitability, exhaustion of the cortical cells, feverish states, and hypertensive crisis.

Typically, Rhodiola rosea is administered in 100 to 150 milligram dosages, 15 to 20 minutes before eating. Larger doses are used in psychiatric treatment (200 milligrams, twice daily) for one to four months.

Modern Western medicine has long since adopted the "one drug—one disease" paradigm; the never-ending search for a "magic bullet" for each illness goes unabated. Eastern medicine practitioners, and more specifically, Chinese medicine practitioners, have based their philosophy on prevention using "harmonizing" remedies for over a thousand years. Today, we know these remedies as adaptogens, and Russia has led the thrust in discovering and using several, including Rhodiola rosea. In fact, Rhodiola rosea's ability to increase the body's ability to "cope" or adapt to physical and psychological stress led the USSR to officially accept it as a medicine as early as 1962. Soviet athletes took Rhodiola rosea regularly in an effort to improve performance, and Soviet scientists recommended it for soldiers and anyone else involved in strenuous physical and mental activity.

The multitude of studies done on Rhodiola rosea make it possible to recommend it for combating tiredness arising during the performance of intense muscular work as well as to accelerate the recovery process. As experiments have shown, Rhodiola transcends its primary use for performance enhancement. So popular is Rhodiola rosea that in the eastern countries, the beverage called "Zlaten tonik Altay" successfully competes with Coca-Cola®.

Rhodiola rosea is truly an adaptogen that has surpassed the expectations of the scientific community. Instead of guzzling coffee for an energy boost, perhaps we should fill our mugs with "Zlaten tonik Altay" or "nastojka" and toast to good health. *Nastrovia!*

CONCLUSION

Rhodiola rosea (Arctic Root)—Not Just Another Adaptogen

Empirical medicine has long extolled the virtues of many herbs for enhancing resistance. Research has demonstrated that many of the benefits attributed to these herbs are due to their adaptogenic properties. Adaptogens have been scientifically reported through clinical and scientific studies for more than 40 years, with their actions well documented and safety confirmed. While ginseng has stolen the spotlight with regard to this category of herbs, the significance and benefits of the Rhodiola rosea plant are beginning to unfold.

It wasn't until 1932 that Dr. L. Utkin, a Russian botanist and nutritionist, performed some of the first research on the plant. In addition to the plant's ability to increase physical endurance, he discovered that the plant increased sexual performance. The use of Rhodiola rosea has a legendary history for increasing health and longevity that has been passed on from generation to generation in Russia. It is said that, "People who drink Rhodiola rosea tea will live more than 100 years."

Rhodiola rosea (arctic root) is not just another adaptogen; this is because it possesses several unique properties that are specific to the plant. These active constituents have been shown to elicit therapeutic efficacy in a diverse collection of conditions. Today, the benefits of Rhodiola rosea go far beyond its adaptogenic activity. Research into these active constituents have demonstrated its versatility in the areas of cardioprotection, anti-cancer activity and antidepressant effects.

Rhodiola rosea is probably the only substance to reach the West in significant quantities which is not claimed to be a cure for anything in particular yet may be an important adjunct to help almost any disease condition. It is also an ideal supplement for healthy people who should take it regularly to increase resistance to disease. This is especially true when an individual is undergoing a period of physical or emotional stress.

These days such herbs are termed adaptogenic—

having the ability to increase the body's ability to cope or adapt to a variety of stresses. Without a doubt, Rhodiola rosea is probably the most successful and versatile of the adaptogens now available.

RESOURCES

Where to Buy Rhodiola rosea

Companies That Sell Rhodiola

1.) Solgar Vitamin & Herb
500 Willow Tree Road
Leonia, New Jersey 07605
Phone (201) 944-2311
Fax (201) 944-7351
Web Site: www.solgar.com

2.) Nature's Plus
548 Broadhollow Road
Melville, New York 11747
Phone (516) 293-0030
Fax (516) 293-0349

3.) Natural Balance
3130 N. Commerce Ct.
Castle Rock, Colorado 80104-8002
Phone (303) 686-6633
Fax (303) 688-1591

4.) Nutraceutical Corporation
1500 Kearns Blvd.
Suite B-200
Park City, Utah 84060
Phone (435) 655-6124
Fax (435) 655-6029

5.) Quest IV Health Products
2352 Greendale Drive
Sarasota, Florida 43232
Phone (941) 342-1250
Fax (941) 342-6085

6.) Carotec
2900 14th Street North
Suite 12
Naples, Florida 33940
Phone (941) 353-2348
Fax (941) 353-2365

Raw Material Supplier of Rhodiola rosea

Pharmline, Inc.
41 Bridge Street
PO Box 291
Florida, New York 10921
Phone (914) 651-4443
Fax (914) 651-6900
Suppliers of Rosavin™ a special standardized form of Rhodiola rosea

REFERENCES

Afanaśeva, S.A., and Alekseeva, E.D., Bardamova, I.B., Maslova, L.V., Lishmanov, Y.B. Cardiac contractile function following acute cooling of the body and the adaptogenic correction of its disorders. *Proceedings of Experimental Biology and Medicine* 116:480–483. Nov Moscow 1993.

Al´Absi, M., Everson, S.A., and Lovallo, W.R. ''Hypertension risk factors and cardiovascular reactivity to mental stress in young men.'' *Int. J. Psychophysiol.* 20(3): 155–60 1995.

American Journal of Medicine, 80: 924–9 1986.

Baranov, V.M. ''Experimental trials of herbal adaptogen effect on the quality of operator activity, mental and professional working capacity.'' Institute of Medical and Biological Problems, Russian Federation Ministry of Health, phase one 1994.

Baranov, V.M. ''Experimental trials of herbal adaptogen effect on the quality of operator activity, mental and professional working capacity.'' Institute of Medical and Biological Problems, Russian Federation Ministry of Health, phase two 1994.

Baranov, V.M. ''The response of cardio-vascular system to dosed physical load under the effect of herbal adaptogen.'' Institute of Medical and Biological Problems, Russian Federation Ministry of Health, phase one 1993–1994.

Baranov, V.M. ''The response of cardio-vascular system to dosed physical load under the effect of herbal adaptogen.'' Institute of Medical and Biological Problems, Russian Federation Ministry of Health, phase two 1993–1994.

Barilyak, I.R., and Dugan, A.M. ''Investigation of antimutagenic effect of alcohol extracts from tissue cultures of Rhodiola rosea and Polyscias in experiments with Salmonella typhimurium.'' *Dopovidi Akademiyi Ukrayiny.* 0(11): 164–167 1994.

Bellmann, K., et al. ''Low stress response enhances vulnerability of islet m-cells in diabetes-prone BB rats.'' *Diabetes.* 46(2): 232–6 1997.

Biondi, M., Costantini, A., and Parisi, A. ''Can loss and grief activate latent neoplasia? A clinical case of possible interaction between genetic risk and stress in breast cancer.'' *Psychother. Psychosom.* 65(2): 102–5 1996.

Blair G.W. 1986. Treatment hypoglycomia. U.S. Patent Office, USA Patent 4602043.

Bocharova. O.A., et al. "The effect of a Rhodiola rosea extract on the incidence of recurrences of superficial bladder cancer." *Urol. Nefrol.* (Mosk), (2): 46–7 1995.

Bolchakova, I.V., Lozoskaya, E.L., and Sapezhinski, I.I. Antioxidant properties of a series of extracts from medicinal plants. *Biophysics,* 42: 1480–1485 1996.

Borovskaia, T.G., Fomina, T.I., and Iaremenko, K.V. A decrease in the toxic action of rubomycin on the small intestine of mice with a transplantable tumor through the use of a Rhodiola extract. *Antibiot Khimioter.* 33(8):615–617 1988.

Breznitz, S., et al. "Experimental induction and termination of acute psychological stress in human volunteers: effects on immunological, neuroendocrine, cardiovascular and psychological parameters." *Brain Behav. Immun.* 12(1): 34–52 1998.

Breivik, T., et al. "Emotional stress effects on immunity, gingivitis and periodontitis." *Eur. J. Oral Sci.* 104(4 (pt 1)): 327–34 1996.

Brosschot, J.F., et al. "Influence of life stress on immunological reactivity to mild psychological stress." *Psychosom. Med.* 56: 216–224 1994.

Bryla, C.M. "The relationship between stress and the development of breast cancer: a literature review." *Oncol. Nurs. Forum.* 23(3): 441–8 1996.

Chen, X.J., et al. Studies of the hypoglycemic effect of Rhodiola sachalinensis A Bor. Polysaccharides. Chung Kuo Chung Yao Tsa Chin. 18: 557–559 1993.

Cholst, S. "Cancer and stress." *Med. Hypotheses.* 46(2): 101–6 1996.

Dantzer, R. "Stress and immunity: what have we learned from psychoneuroimmunology?" *Acta Physiol. Scand. Suppl.* 640(): 43–6 1997.

Davis, L.L., Suris, A., and Lambert, M.T. Heimberg, C., Petty, F. "Post-traumatic stress disorder and serotonin: new directions for research and treatment." *J. Psychiatry Neurosci.* 22(5): 318–26 1997.

Dement´eva, L.A., and Iaremenko, K.V. Effect of a *Rhodiola* extract on the tumor process in an experiment. *Vopr Onkol,* 33(7): 57–60 1987.

Dement´eva, L.A., and Iaremenko, K.V. The study of the influence of Rhodiola rosea extract on the growth of tumors in experiment. Proceedings of Siberian Department of the USSR Academy of Science, 6: 70–77 1983.

Dhabhar, F.S., and McEwen, B.S. "Acute stress enhances while chronic stress suppresses cell-mediated immunity in vivo: a potential role for leukocyte trafficking." *Brain Behav. Immun.* 11(4): 286–306 1997.

Dreher, D., and Junod, A.F. "Role of oxygen free radicals in cancer development." *Eur. J. Cancer.* 32A(1): 30–8 1996.

Drummond, P.D., Hewson-Bower, B. "Increased psychological stress and decreased mucosal immunity in children with recurrent upper respiratory tract infections." *J. Psychosom. Res.* 43(3): 271–8 1997.

References

Dutour, A., et al. ''Hormonal response to stress in brittle diabetes.'' *Psychoneuroendicrinology,* 21(6): 525–43 1996.

Eliot, R.S. ''Stress and the heart. Mechanisms, measurements and management.'' *Postgrad. Med.* 92(5): 237–42, 245–8 1992.

Evans, S.J., Levi, A.J., and Jones, J.V. ''Wall stress induced arrhythmia is enhanced by low potassium and early left ventricular hypertrophy in the working rat heart.'' *Cardiovasc. Res.* 29(4): 555–62 1995.

Fichtner, C.G., et al. ''Hypodensity of platelet serotonin uptake sites in posttraumatic stress disorder. Associated clinical features.'' *Life Sci.* 57(2): PL37–44 1995.

Fleming, L. Parkinson's disease and brain levels of organochlorines pesticides. *Ann. Neurol.* 36: 100–103 1994.

Fontana, F., et al. ''Pressor effects of endogenous opioid system during acute episodes of blood pressure increases in hypertensive patients.'' *Hypertension.* 29(1): 105–110 1997.

Francis, R.A., et al. ''The relationship of blood pressure to a brief measure of anger during routine health screening.'' *J. Natl. Med. Assoc.* 83(7): 1–4 1991.

Frolova, G.I., et al. Use of a Golden root *(Rhodiola rosea)* tincture in training periodontosis. *Stomatology* 60: 81–82. Moscow 1981.

Goranchuk, V.V., and Smirnov, V.S. ''Patterns of the changes in the indices of B-system immunity in acute psychoemotional stress.'' *Med. Tr. Prom. Ekol.* (4): 19–22 1995.

References

Hassig, A., Liang, W.X., and Stampfli, K. "Stress-induced suppression of the cellular immune reactions. A contribution on the neuroendocrine control of the immune system." *Med. Hyp.* 46: 551–5 1996.

Helmers, K.F., et al. "Stress and depressed mood in medical students, law students and graduate students at McGill University." *Acad. Med.* 72(8): 708–14 1997.

Hirota, M., et al. "Effects of hypokalaemia on arrhythmogenic risk of quinidine in rats" Life Sci, 62(24): 159–69 1998.

Holm, E., et al. "Linkage between post-absorptive amino acid release and glutamate uptake in skeletal muscle tissue of healthy young subjects, cancer patients and the elderly." *J. Mol. Med.* 75(6): 454–61 1997.

Iakubovskii, M., et al. The activity of the lipid peroxidation processes in the mucosa of the rat small intestine and its morpho-functional state under acute irradiation and the administration of combined preparations created on a base of highly dispersed silica. *Radiation Biology and Radio-ecology,* 37(3): 366–71 May–Jun 1997.

Jern, S., Bergbrant, A., Hedner, T., and Hansson, L. "Enhanced pressor responses to experimental and daily-life stress in borderline hypertension." *J. Hypertens.* 13(1): 69–79 1995.

Kang, S. Zhang, J., Lu, Y., and Lu, D. Chemical constituents of *Rhodiola kirilowii* (Reg.) Institute of Qinghai High Altitude Medical Scientific Research, Xining. Chung Kuo Chung Yao Tsa Chih, 17(2): 100–1, 127 Feb 1992.

References

Kanno, J., et al. "Effect of restraint stress on immune system and experimental B16 melanoma metastasis in aged mice." *Mech. Aging Dev.*, 93(1–3): 107–17 1997.

Khushbatove, Z.A., et al. "Study of the lypolipidemic properties of polymer proanthocyanidins from plants used in folk medicine." *Pharm. J.* 23(9): 111–1115 1989.

Khnykina, L.A., and Zotova, M.I. To the pharmacognostic study of Rhodiola rosea. *Apthech. Delo* 15: 34–38 1996.

Komar, V.V., et al. Macro- and microelement composition of root extracts of *Rhodiola rosea. Pharm. J.* 3: 58–60 Jun 1980.

Krendall, F.P., et al. "Examining the hepatoprotective effect of a preparation made from Rhodiola rosea culture biomass." *Farmatsiya.* 44(3): 35–8 1995.

Kurkin, V.A., and Zapesochnaya, G.G. Chemical composition and pharmacological properties of *Rhodiola rosea. Chem. and Pharm. J.* Moscow 20 (10): 1231–44 1986.

Kurmukov, A.G.; Aizikov, M.I., and Rakhimov, S.S. Pharmacology of the plant polyphenol epigalokhin. *Farmakol Toksikol,* 49(2):45–8 1986 Mar–Apr.

Laaris, N., et al. "Stress-induced alterations of somatodendritic 5–HT1A autoreceptor sensitivity in the rat dorsal raphe nucleus—in vitro electrophysiological evidence." *Fundam. Clin. Pharmacol.* 11(3): 206–14 1997.

Lazarova, M.B., et al. Effects of meclofenoxate and Extr. *Rhodiolae roseae* L. on electroconvulsive shock-impaired learning and memory in rats. *Meth. Find Exp. Clin. Pharmacol.* 8(9): 547–52 Sept 1986.

Lee, D., Lu, Z.W., and DeQuattro, V. "Neural mechanisms in primary hypertension. Efficacy of alpha-blockade with doxazosin during stress." *Am. J. Hypertens.* 9(1): 47–53 1996.

Li, T., et al. "Repeated restraint stress impairs the anti-tumor T cell response through its suppressive effect on Th1–type CD4+ cells." *Anticancer Res.* 17(6D): 4259–68 1997.

Lishmanov, Iu.B., et al. "Contribution of the opioid system to realization of inotropic effects of Rhodiola rosea extracts in ischemic and reperfusion heart damage in vitro." *Eksp. Klin. Farmakol.* 60(3): 34–6 1997.

Lishmanov, Iu.B., et al. The anti-arrhythmia effect of Rhodiola rosea and its possible mechanism." *Biull. Eksp. Biol. Med.* 116(8): 175–6 1993 Aug.

Lishmanov, Iu.B., et al. Plasma beta-endorphin and stress hormones in stress and adaptation. *Biull. Eksp. Biol. Med.* 103(4): 422–4 1987 Apr 1987.

L'opez, J.F., et al. "A.E. Bennett Award. Regulation of serotonin1A, glucocorticoid and mineralcorticoid receptor in rat and human hippocampus: implications for the neurobiology of depression." *Biol. Psychiatry.* 43(8): 547–73 1998.

Mahboob, T., et al. "Stress and hypertension: role of serum, red cell and tissue electrolytes." *Life Sci.* 58(18): 1587-90 1996.

Maimeshkulova, L.A., et al. The participation of the mu-, delta- and kappa-opioid receptors in the realization of the anti-arrhythmia effect of Rhodiola rosea. *Experi.* and Clini. *Pharmacop.* Moscow 60: 38–9 1997.

Marina, T.F., Alekseeva, L.P., and Plotnikova, T.M. The influence of *Rhodiola rosea* preparation on the spontaneous bioelectric activity and electrographic reactions of the cortex of the large hemispheres and some subcortical structures. Proceedings of Siberian Department of the USSR Academy of Science. *Biol. Sci.* 3: 85–9 1973.

Maslov, L.N., et al. "Mechanism of the anti-arrhythmic effect of the Rhodiola rosea extract." *Biull. Eksp. Biol. Med.* 125(4): 424–6 1998.

Maslova, L.V., et al. The cardioprotective and antiadrenergic activity of an extract of *Rhodiola rosea* in stress. *Exper. and Clin. Pharmacol.*, 57(6):61–3 1994 Nov–Dec 1994.

McCormack, K.J., and Chapleo, C.B. "Opioid receptors and myocardial protection." *Clin Drug Invest,* 15(5): 445-454 1998

McNaughton, M.E., et al. "The relationship among stress, depression, locus of control, irrational beliefs, social support and health in Alzheimer's disease caregivers." *J. Nerv. Ment. Dis.* 183(2): 78–85 1995.

Miller, J.W., Selhub, J., and Joseph, J.A. "Oxidative damage caused by free radicals produced during catecholamine autoxidation: protective effects of O-methylation and melatonin." *Free Radic. Biol. Med.* 21(2): 241–9 1996.

Molokovskii, D.S., Davydov, V.V., and Tiulenev, V.V. The action of adaptogenic plant preparations in experimental alloxan diabetes. *Probl Endo.* Moscow, 35(6): 82–7 Nov–Dec. 1989.

Munck, A., Guyre, P.M., Holbrook, N.J. ''Physiological functions of glucocorticoids in stress and their relation to pharmacological actions'' *Endocr. Rev.* 5(1): 25–44 1984.

Naliboff, B.D., et al. ''The effects of the opiate antagonist naloxone on measures of cellular immunity during rest and brief psychological stress.'' *J. Psychosom. Res.* 39(3): 345–59 1995.

Peng, J.N., Ma, C.Y., and Ge, Y.C. Chemical constituents of *Rhodiola kirilowii* (Regel) Regel. Chung Kuo Chung Yao Tsa Chih, 19(11): 676–7, 702 Nov 1994.

Perna, F.M., Schneiderman, N. and LaPerriere, A. ''Psychological stress, exercise and immunity.'' *Int. J. Sports Med.* 18Suppl 1(): S78–83 1997.

Petkov, V.D., et al. Effects of alcohol aqueous extract from *Rhodiola rosea* L. roots on learning and memory. *Acta. Physiol. Pharmacol. Bulg.* 12(1): 3–16 1986.

Polozny, A.V., et al. *Rhodiola rosea* or Golden root. Biology of Siberian plants requiring protection. *Novosibirsk* 85–114 1985.

Porta, C., et al. ''Antioxidant enzymatic system and free radicals pathway in two different human cancer cells.'' *Anticancer Res.* 16(5A): 2741–7 1996.

Saratikov, A.S. Golden Root *(Rhodiola rosea). Tomsk,* p. 155 1974.

Saratikov, A.S., and Krasnov, E.A. *Rhodiola rosea* is a valuable Medicinal Plant. *Tomsk,* p. 252.

Saratikov, A.S., Salnik, B.U., and Revina, T.A. Biochemical Characteristics of the Stimulative Action of Rodosine during prescribed Muscular Workloads. Proceedings of Siberian Department of Academy of Sciences of the USSR. *Biol. Sci.* 5: 108–115 1968.

Saratikov, A.S., et al. Rhodiolosid, a new glycosid from *Rhodiola rosea* and its pharmacological properties. *Pharmazie* 23: 392–5 1968.

Salikhova, R.A., et al. ''Effect of Rhodiola rosea on the yield of mutation alterations and DNA repair in bone marrow cells.'' *Patol. Fiziol. Eksp. Ter.* (4): 22–4 1997.

Schedlowski, M., and Schmidt, R.E. ''Stress and the immune system.'' *Naturwissenschaften.* 83(5): 214–20 1996.

Schultz, J.E., Hsu, A.K., and Gross, G.J. ''Morphine mimics the cardio-protective effect of ischemic preconditioning via a glibenclamide-sensitive mechanism in the rat heart.'' *Circ. Res.* 78(6): 1100–4 1996.

Schultz, J.J., Hsu, A.K., and Gross, G.J. ''Ischemic preconditioning and morphine-induced cardio-protection involve the delta-opioid receptor in the intact rat heart.'' *J. Mol. Cell. Cardiol.* 29(8): 2187–95 1997.

Schultz, J.E., et al. ''Evidence for involvement of opioid receptors in ischemic preconditioning in rat hearts.'' *Am. J. Physiol.* 268(5 pt 2): H2157–61 1995.

Seaton, K.E., D.Sc., and Micozzi, M., M.D, Ph.D. ''Is cortisol the aging hormone?'' *J. Adv. Med.* 11(2) 1998.

Sheridan, J.F. ''Norman Cousins Memorial Lecture 1997. Stress-induced modulation of anti-viral immunity.'' *Brain Behav. Immun.* 12(1): 1–6 1998.

Singh, N., et al. ''Psychological stress and depression in older patients with intravenous drug use and human immunodeficiency virus infection: implications for intervention.'' *Int. J. STD AIDS.* 8(4): 251–5 1997.

Skurygin, V.P. ''Reverse absorption of serotonin by synaptosomes and its level in the rat cerebral cortex in acute and chronic stress.'' *Vopr. Med.* Khim, 41(3): 39–41 1995.

Sommers–Flanagan, J., Greenberg, R.P. ''Psychosocial variables and hypertension: a new look at an old controversy.'' *J. Nerv. Ment. Dis.* 177(1): 15–24 1989.

Spiridonov, N.A., and Arkhipov, V.V. ''Cytostatic action of medicinal plants on cultured lymphoblastoids.'' *KhimikoFarmatsevticheskii Zhurnal,* 28(9): 49–51 1994.

Sprouse, J.S. and Aghajanian, G.K. ''Electrophysiological responses of serotoninergic dorsal raphe neurons to 5HT1A and 5HT1B agonists.'' *Synapse.* 1: 3–9 1987.

Starkey, S.J. and Skingle M. "5HT1D as well as 5HT1A autoreceptors modulate 5HT release in the guinea pig dorsal raphe nucleus" *Neuropharmacol.* 33: 393–402 1994.

Strausbaugh, H., and Irwin, M. "Central corticotropinreleasing hormone reduces cellular immunity." *Brain Behav. Immun.* 6(1): 11–7 1992.

Takao T., Hashimoto K., DeSouza E.B. "Modulation of interleukin-1 receptors in the brain-endocrine-immune axis by stress and infection." *Brain Behav. Immun.*, 9(4): 276-91 1995.

Turnbull B.S., Cowan D.F. "Myocardial contraction band necrosis in stranded cetaceans." *J. Comp. Pathol.*, 118(4): 317-27 1998.

Udintsev, S.N., and Shakhov, V.P. Decrease in the growth rate of Ehrlich's tumor and Pliss' lymphosarcoma with partial hepatectomy. *Vopr. Onkol.* 35(9): 1072–5 1989.

Udintsev, S.N., and Shakhov, V.P. Changes in clonogenic properties of bone marrow and transplantable mice tumor cells during combined use of cyclophosphane and biological response modifiers of adaptogenic origin. *Eksp. Onkol.* 12(6):55–56 1990.

Udintsev, S.N., and Shakhov, V.P. The role of humoral factors of regenerating liver in the development of experimental tumors and the effect of Rhodiola rosea extract on this process. *Neoplasma* 38(3): 323–31 1991.

Udintsev, S.N., Shakhov, V.P., and Borovskoi, I.G. Mechanism of differential effect of low dose adaptogens on the functional activity of normal and transformed cellular elements in vitro. *Biofizika.* 36(4):624–7 Jul–Aug 1991.

Udintsev, S.N., et al. The effect of low concentrations of adaptogen solutions on the functional activity of murine bone marrow cells in vitro. *Biofizika.* 36(1): 105–8 Jan–Feb 1991.

Udintsev, S.N., Krylova, S.G., and Fomina, T.I. The enhancement of the efficacy of adriamycin by using hepatoprotectors of plant origin in metastases of Ehrlich's adenocarcinoma to the liver in mice. *Vopr. Onkol.* 38(10):1217–22 1992.

Viner, R., McGrath, M., and Trudinger, P. "Family stress and metabolic control in diabetes." *Arch. Dic. Child.* 74(5): 418–21 1996.

Wales J.K. "Does psychological stress cause diabetes?" *Diabet. Med.,* 12(2): 109-12 1995.

Walker, Q.D., and Mailman, R.B. Triadimefon and triadimenol: effects on monoamine uptake and release. *Toxicol. Appl. Pharmacol.* 139: 2, 227–33 Aug 1996.

Wang, S., and Wang, F.P. Studies on the chemical components of *Rhodiola* crenulata. Department of Chemistry of Natural Medicinal Products, College of Pharmacy, West China University of Medical Sciences, Chengdu. *Yao Hsueh Hsueh Pao.* 27(2): 117–20 1992.

Wang, S. You, X.T., and Wang, F.P. HPLC determination of salidroside in the roots of *Rhodiola* genus plants. College of Pharmacy, West China University of Medical Sciences, Chengdu. *Yao Hsueh Hsueh Pao.* 27(11): 849–52 1992.

Westly, H.J., and Kelley, K.W. "Physiologic concentrations of cortisol suppress cell-mediated immune events in the domestic pig." *Proc. Soc. Exp. Biol. Med.* 177(1): 156–64 1984.

Xiang, S., and Zhao, H. "Interrelationship between magnesium and potassium in preventing myocardial ischemia reperfusion arrhythmia." *Chin. Med. J.* 109(4): 282–5 1996.

Yoshikawa, M., et al. Rhodiocyanosides A and B, new antiallergic cyanoglycosides from Chinese natural medicine "si lie hong jing tian," the underground part of *Rhodiola quadrifida* (Pall.) Fisch. et Mey. *Chem. Pharm. Bull.* (Tokyo), 43(7): 1245-7 Jul 1995.

Yoshikawa, M., et al. Bioactive constituents of Chinese natural medicines. II. *Rhodiola radix.* (1). Chemical structures and antiallergic activity of rhodiocyanosides A and B from the underground part of Rhodiola quadrifida (Pall) Fisch et Mey. (Crassulaceae). *Chem. Pharm. Bull.* (Tokyo). 44 (11): 2086–91 1996.

Zhang, Z.H., et al. Effect of *Rhodiola Maxim* on preventing high altitude reactions. A comparison of cardiopulmonary function in villagers at various altitudes. *Chung Kuo Chung Yao Tsa Chih* 14(11): 687–90, 704 Nov 1989.

Zhang, Z., et al. Electron microscopic observation of the effects of *Rhodiola kirilowii* (Regel.) Maxim. In preventing damage of the rat viscera by a hypoxic high altitude environment. *Chung Kuo Chung Yao Tsa Chih.* 15(3):177–81, 192 Mar 1990.

Zhang, S., Wang, J., and Zhang, H. Chemical constituents of Tibetan medicinal herb Rhodiola kirilowii (Reg.) Reg.*Gansu Chung Kuo Chung Yao Tsa Chih,* 16(8): 483, 512 Aug 1991.

Zehender, M., et al. ''Anti-arrhythmic effects of increasing the daily intake of magnesium and potassium in patients with frequent ventricular arrhythmias. Magnesium in cardiac arrhythmias investigators.'' J Am Coll Cardiol, 29 (5): 1028–34 1997.

ABOUT THE AUTHORS

Carl Germano, R.D., C.N.S., L.D.N., is a registered and certified clinical nutritionist and practitioner of Chinese herbology. He holds a master's degree in clinical nutrition from New York University and has over twenty years of experience using innovative, complementary nutritional therapy in private practice. For the past twelve years, he has dedicated his efforts to research and product development for the dietary supplement industry, where he has been instrumental in bringing cutting-edge nutritional substances and formulations to the market. Presently, he is vice president of product development with the Solgar Vitamin & Herb company. Today, he continues his efforts in product development and research and is responsible for providing the dietary supplement industry with the next generation of clinically important nutritional substances. Mr. Germano is Adjunct Professor of Nutrition at New York Chiropractic College, as well as a frequent radio guest and columnist on the subject of nutrition. Additionally, he is the author of *The Osteoporosis Solution* and coauthor of *The Brain Wellness Plan.*

Zakir Ramazanov, Ph.D., is a professor of plant biochemistry and has authored more than 130 scientific articles and patents in the field of biotechnology, plant biochemistry, and molecular biology. Dr. Ramazanov has served as a professor at The Technological Institute, Las Palmas, Spain, and as Senior Scientist at the Russian Academy of Science. His achievements include his position as Scientific Coordinator of Algal Biotechnology and his work in space biology and cultivation of photosynthetic organisms in space stations. Presently, he is the executive vice president of scientific affairs at Pharmline, Inc.

Dr. Maria del Mar Bernal Suarez is director of the Technical Services Department at Pharmline Inc. She obtained her Ph.D. at the University of Las Palmas, Spain. She identified the most important key active constituents in Arctic root, and she developed Rosavin™—Pharmline's standardized extract of Rhodiola rosea. Her unique experience in analytical chemistry made possible the identification and introduction of genetically true and clinically researched species of Rhodiola rosea in the U.S.